HELPING YOURSELF WITH HOMEOPATHIC REMEDIES

D1328905

A Doctor's Guide to
HELPING YOURSELF
WITH
HOMEOPATHIC
REMEDIES

by

JAMES H. STEPHENSON, M.D.

THORSONS PUBLISHERS LIMITED
Wellingborough, Northamptonshire

First published in the United Kingdom 1977
Sixth Impression 1983

*Original American edition published by
Parker Publishing Company, West Nyack, New York*

© PARKER PUBLISHING COMPANY INC. 1976

ISBN 0 7225 0372 5

Printed and bound in Great Britain

What This Book Can Do for You

You have used homeopathy all your life! Simply stated, we treat ourselves homeopathically if, when we are ill, we take a substance that would produce our symptoms in a healthy person. An everyday example is the old home remedy (used particularly among Italian-Americans) of raw onions or garlic for a cold. These work homeopathically because they produce in healthy people the sneezing, running eyes and nose, and itching and burning discharge of a cold.

Probably our first connection with homeopathy was a smallpox vaccination or diptheria-pertussus-tetanus immunization. In each instance we took a substance (like tetanus antitoxin) in order to prevent later illness. Or, those of us who have had hangovers know that a "hair of the dog that bit you" often makes the world livable again. Or, if you ever had to live in a tropical climate without the benefits of air conditioning you know—as the English discovered when they occupied India—that cold drinks can bring on heat convulsion and apoplexy but *hot* drinks can help you survive. Equally, to tolerate the rigors of a cold climate the English start the day with a cold bath and the Finns take a hot air sauna and then roll in the snow or cut a hole in the ice.

In each of these examples the treatment—such as alcohol or heat or cold—could produce the troubles in the first place.

Likewise, any time we receive quinine for malaria, colchicine for gout, or X-ray for skin cancer we are treated by an agent which would produce our symptoms in the healthy.

Thus, there's nothing mysterious about homeopathy! Rather, it has always been an unrecognized part of our lives.

Certainly, homeopathy is not the only way of treating illness. But it has a wide application and makes possible the relief of diseases that would not respond any other way.

Homeopathic medicines are specially prepared dilutions of natural substances, largely herbs. For instance, the common herbs *Chamomile* and *Ipecac* are available from homeopathic pharmacies in specially diluted form. Also, many natural mineral, animal, reptile, insect and bacterial products have been tested and prepared for homeopathic use. With over 2,000 specially prepared, highly effective medicines at his disposal, the homeopathic physician is well equipped to treat most common, and many uncommon illnesses.

Homeopathic physicians are medical specialists. Membership in the various state and national homeopathic organizations is open *only* to licensed physicians. Like all medical specialties, homeopathic therapy is a complex and difficult subject, requiring years of supervised study.

Homeopathy can treat most illnesses, ranging from mild colds to serious diseases like pneumonia, providing at the least a safe, cheap starting point for treatment. This book tells you how to treat yourself homeopathically for literally dozens of conditions. You will find whole sections devoted to respiratory diseases such as influenza and the common cold, digestive tract upsets such as colitis and constipation, bone and joint diseases such as arthritis, female troubles such as painful menses or complaints from the menopause, nervous troubles such as depression or the bad effects of grief and separation, skin troubles such as hives and eczema, heart disease such as heart failure, and allergies such as hay fever and food sensitivities.

If you are concerned about a particular health problem you can probably find it in the index at the end of the book, referring to the appropriate section for its treatment. Please understand that because this is a book on home treatment for persons without any medical training, all our discussions just scratch the surface of possible homeopathic treatment for your condition. But even with this limitation you may be amazed at the results you can achieve!

All homeopathic medicines were first tested on healthy persons. This is a guarantee of their safety and effectiveness. Since the tests are recorded in everyday language, not medical terms, this method provides a *people-oriented medicine.* Therefore, homeopathic medicines can treat *all* our complaints, not just our illnesses.

Homeopathic medicines treat the whole person. Because the homeopathic medicines are first tested on healthy persons and the effects noted in the everyday language of these healthy persons, the full range of medicine action—subjective as well as objective, emotional and mental as well as physical—is recorded and is therefore available for treating your own physical, emotional and mental symptoms totally. Thus, a single homeopathic medicine is often able to relieve a whole number of your physical, emotional and mental complaints at once.

Homeopathy treats people, not just diseases. We each get sick differently. One person with the flu will be chilly, another hot, one will ache all over, another will be nauseated. Homeopathic treatment has a separate medicine for each of these types of flu. Thus, treatment is *individualized* to the patient. As you will see later on in this book, part of the challenge and downright fun of homeopathy is finding the particular "medicine-picture" that fits your particular illness!

Subjective symptoms are vital for homeopathic treatment. Our outer, objective symptoms such as skin rashes or discolorations are readily visible to other persons. Not so, however, with our inner, subjective symptoms such as our experience of pain, our fears and joys, etc. These subjective symptoms are necessarily private for each of us and remain so unless we tell other persons of their presence. The homeopathic physician nearly always includes your subjective symptoms in his evaluation. This helps him understand your individual reaction to your particular troubles, as it is usually our subjective reactions which define our personal individualities.

Homeopathy can treat generally unrecognized conditions. Sometimes we just feel rotten without having an identifiable illness. We *know* we're sick and we don't want to be told it's our imagination! Homeopathy has medications for these "non-disease" miseries. No longer do you have to fit into some disease picture to "qualify" for treatment. Because your total subjective symptoms, stated in your own words, are the basis for your homeopathic treatment, individual problems unique to *you* may be relieved. For example, some people feel miserable on waking and drag around half-dead until noon. That's not a disease but it can really louse up a person's life, particularly if he has to function properly in the morning. Well, homeopathy has dozens of medicines for this condition. Or, some of us are so hypersensitive to our surroundings that the least sound, or odor or change of temperature or atmospheric condition will make us unhappy, angry, inefficient or, even, physically sick. Homeopathy has dozens of medicines for this, as well as for hundreds of other individual symptom-reaction patterns that are not generally recognized as "acceptable" illnesses.

We all have great abilities for self-healing. On examination after death persons are often found to have lived with or to have recovered from illnesses of which they had never been aware. As a result, many scientists believe we are constantly repairing (or walling off when repair is impossible) unhealthy cells and tissues. In this manner, we have all overcome—probably frequently overcome—illnesses such as polio, cancer, tuberculosis, pneumonia, etc., etc. From this viewpoint, we only become sick when we have lost this ability for self-repair. Certain amphibians, like the salamander, can even regenerate whole new limbs.

Homeopathic medicines cooperate with our own self-healing. As a result, just the way a good spring housecle ning gets the dirt out from under the rug, homeopathic medicines may often bring back old, unresolved problems so they can be relieved. Or they may move an illness from a vital to a less vital part as the sudden appearance of a rash on the chest after a cough has disappeared. Or they may bring your problem to a head in order to get rid of it quickly.

Therefore, if after you have taken a few drops or a pinch of a homeopathic medicine your immediate problem gets momentarily worse, or if it gets better but seems to move to a less vital part, or if old problems momentarily reappear, do not be alarmed! These are all good signs that the homeopathic medicine is helping your body "clean house." And do not use any non-homeopathic medicines or treatments of any kind as they may push your troubles back in, interfering with your own self-healing. Do not even repeat the homeopathic medicine at this point as that may also interfere. Just leave yourself alone so your own self-healing abilities can finish the job!

Homeopathic medicines are usually made into specially energized high dilutions, completely different from other types of medicines. One part of the original medicine substance is added to nine parts of a diluting substance such as ethyl alcohol in water, or milk sugar. This mixture is agitated many times and one part of it is diluted with nine parts of a fresh substance and agitated again. When the process has been repeated six times you have a 6th decimal dilution (called the 6x dilution by homeopathic pharmacists). Twelve repetitions produces a 12th decimal or 12x dilution. For convenience, these liquid dilutions are often put in grains or tablets of milk sugar.

Although the simple undiluted alcoholic tinctures are sometimes used by homeopathic physicians, many medicines become safe only if diluted. Therefore, I suggest you limit your home treatment efforts to the 6x or 12x dilutions. Of course, even higher dilutions are available from homeopathic pharmacists but they are only suitable for use by physicians.

As homeopathic pharmacies are too few, you may sometimes wish to make your own home medicines. A quick way to "roll your own" medicine is to start with a small container of a water or alcohol dilution of the substance you wish to make into a medicine. Empty this container (enough medicine clings to its walls to start the next dilution) and refill it with the diluting liquid. Strike the container fifteen times against the palm of your hand. Empty, and repeat the whole process six or twelve times, producing a 6x or 12x dilution, a drop of which, on your tongue, may give you relief.

Amazingly enough, these homemade medicines are often highly effective. But, after all, that's how homeopathic physicians made their own medicines 100 years ago, before the development of our modern pharmacies. Botanical medicines such as common onion (*Alium cepa*) are particularly easy to prepare at home as their crushed leaves and flowers are usually alcohol-soluble. Water-soluble substances such as salt and sugar also are easily made into home remedies but insoluble substances such as sand must be ground up with milk sugar, step by step, a process too complex for home preparation. Other than your garden and kitchen, the local drugstore may provide other raw materials, such as syrup of Ipecac, for your home-brewed medicines.

At appropriate places throughout this book, you will be told of medicines which you can prepare at home, should you care to do so.

The method of preparing medicines for homeopathic treatment may seem strange or even unnecessary. This specific method of preparation seeks to "free-up" the healing energies in the medicines. Thus the alcoholic tinctures work more safely and many inert substances, such as sand, which have no medicinal action undiluted, develop profound healing properties when diluted.

Recent research, using the most up-to-date equipment, has shown that homeopathic medicines, like the battery in your flashlight, act as *carriers of energy* rather than as chemical drugs. Therefore, they act differently than ordinary medicines, stimulating you to heal yourself, rather than chemically altering your body fluids.

Homeopathic medicines are usually taken by mouth in small doses consisting of a pinch of the granules, or one or two tablets, given once. If there is no reaction in half an hour, you may repeat the medicine twice at half hourly intervals. If there is no effect, that particular medicine is discontinued, or changed to another kind. Because homeopathic medicines are *energy-activators* of your own healing abilities, rather than *chemical antagonists* of your disease, their effect is not related to the size of a dose, a pinch acting as well as a cupful. Because the *amount* you take each time does not matter, obviously the smaller dose you take, the longer your bottle of medicine will last. A convenient amount is a drop of liquid medicine, a pinch of powder or a single tablet in another form.

Homeopathic medicines are pleasant, painless, and convenient to apply. They are prepared in many forms. Most frequently, they consist of pleasant tasting milk sugar tablets or granules. These are taken dry on the tongue, without any food or drinks for 15 minutes before and after. They are also available as ointments or creams, or as solutions for injection by needle. You needn't go to a hospital or any other special place to use the medicine.

Homeopathic medicines are safe, rarely producing toxic side reactions, probably because of their special, highly-dilute, energy-carrying form, and their administration on the similar principle—both producing a natural, supportive action in disease rather than a chemical onslaught. Thus, they offer you a safe beginning for treatment, allowing you to defer potentially dangerous medicines or always dangerous surgery until you have exhausted natural, harmless forms of treatment such as homeopathy, dietary adjustment, manipulation, massage, hot and cold water packs, exercise, rest, etc.

In this manner, homeopathic treatment is a useful supplement for all other forms of treatment. As homeopathic physicians are trained in all types of medical therapy, they can advise their patients whether simple, cheap and safe homeopathic treatment is suitable for them or whether they need to have some other form of treatment.

Homeopathic treatment is cheap. Because they are given in high dilutions and in small, infrequent doses, homeopathic medicines are cheap both to manufacture and administer. As they do not spoil, a typical one dram bottle of homeopathic tablets, costing three to four dollars, may last for years. Also, since homeopathic treatment does not require expensive laboratory tests or hospital treatment, the major cost of medical care is eliminated.

Homeopathic treatment can start immediately as it is based on your total symptoms stated in your own words, not on laboratory tests. In this manner, illnesses can be caught in their early stages, preventing complications both to yourself and your pocketbook! You would be wise to order an assortment of homeopathic medicines before you need them, as mail orders usually take at least one to two months. Many homeopathic pharmacies have home treatment kits already available for order.

Homeopathic medicines are ideal for home treatment as they are safe, gentle, pleasant-tasting, cheap, painless, naturally stimulative, and good for most illnesses and for all the members of your family (including the pets!)

Homeopathic Pharmacies and Bookstores

Homeopathic medicines may be obtained from the sources which follow. I suggest you write to the nearest ones for their catalogues (often provided free): Boericks & Runyon, Div. (Boericke and Tafel), 1011 Arch Street, Philadelphia 19107; Ehrhart & Karl, Inc., 17 North Wabash Avenue, Chicago, Illinois 60602; Luyties

Pharmacal Company, 4200 Laclede Avenue, St. Louis, Missouri 63108; Humphries Medicine Co., Inc., 63 Meadow Rd., Rutherford, New Jersey; Kiehl's Pharmacy, 109 Third Avenue, New York City; Standard Homeopathic Company, 204 West 131 St., Los Angeles, California 90061; Washington Homeopathic Pharmacy, 724-11th Street, N.W., Washington, D.C. 20001; John A. Borneman & Sons, 1208 Amosland Rd., Norwood, Pa. 19074. Unfortunately, the preparation of homeopathic medicines requires special training and equipment, so that the ordinary pharmacy is not usually suited for their preparation. Home treatment kits especially made for this book are available through Similia, Inc., P.O. Box 175, Glenville Station, Conn. 06830.

Homeopathic books may be purchased from: Boericke & Tafel, Inc., 1011 Arch Street, Philadelphia, Pennsylvania 19107; Ehrhart & Karl, Inc., 17 North Wabash Avenue, Chicago, Illinois 60602; Similia, Inc., P.O. Box 175, Glenville Station, Conn. 06830.

Sources of Homeopathic Information

Information about homeopathy is available from various sources. The American Foundation for Homeopathy at 6231 Leesburg Pike, Suite 506, Falls Church, Va. 22044 publishes a magazine, *The Layman Speaks,* and offers a qualifying course in homeopathic treatment for lay persons. It also sponsors local groups entitled "Homeopathic Laymen's Leagues" in many of the larger cities in this country. The Foundation also sponsors a postgraduate summer school of homeopathic instruction for licensed physicians of this country and Canada. It also has a series of pamphlets on homeopathy.

The American Institute of Homeopathy, which shares the same address as the American Foundation for Homeopathy, is the professional organization of homeopathic physicians in the United States. The Institute offers postgraduate tutorials in Homeopathy in the major cities in this country. Through its information arm, The Homeopathic Information Service, it offers pamphlets on homeopathy specifically oriented to physcians and other enquiring scientists and scholars.

Dangers of Casual Homeopathic Treatment

This book attempts to present a difficult medical specialty in a simple form for home use. If it achieves this purpose I shall be grateful. However, do not let its simplicity make you overconfident. *You are not qualified to treat difficult, constitutional cases of illness in yourself or in others.* Any condition which does not quickly show some improvement, particularly if it is life threatening, should be referred to a physician's care. Also, remember that, often, the most difficult cases for a homeopathic physician to unravel are persons who have treated themselves casually, and ignorantly, with partially-indicated homeopathic medicines, over a period of years. In homeopathy, as in most areas of life, a little knowledge may truly be worse than none at all.

James H. Stephenson, M.D.

U.K. Publisher's Note

In the U.K. homeopathic medicines and accessories can be obtained from the following:

A. Nelson & Co., 73 Duke Street, London W1M 6BY

E. Gould & Sons, 67 Moorgate, London EC2

Kilburn Chemists Ltd., 21 Belsize Road, London NW6

The Galen Pharmacy, 1 South Terrace, South Street, Dorchester

Freemans, 7 Eaglesham Road, Clarkston, Glasgow

Further information about homeopathy can be supplied on request by The British Homeopathic Association, 27a Devonshire Street, London W1N 1RJ.

We also publish a growing list of homeopathic books, and details of these can be obtained by writing to Thorsons Publishers Limited, Denington Estate, Wellingborough, Northamptonshire.

Contents

SECTION I
THE GUIDE

1

Tested Homeopathic Remedies for Stomach and Bowel Troubles

Importance of Healthy Intestines

Although most of us have never stopped to consider it, we are literally a walking set of intestines—30 feet of them in the average adult! If you add to this the two feet of stomach and food tube or esophagus leading from our intestines to our mouth, and the two feet of urinary apparatus that deals with the watery end of food digestion, it's no wonder so much of our lives are spent in service to our own digestive systems!

Our first few months mostly all we thought about was food. Indeed, although in this country we're lucky enough to have a superabundance of food, if at any time one of us can't get enough food, for one reason or another, it's still hard to think about anything else. During World War II when I was a prisoner of war I used to dream about food! Although fliers were notorious woman chasers, as we became hungrier our conversation shifted more and more from the pleasures of sex to the pleasures of food. I began to understand why many religious orders keep their celibate priests lean and hungry!

Intestinal Symptoms of Many Diseases Calling for Treatment

Just as our intestines play such an important role in our lives during health, equally so, they participate in most of our diseases. Usually, in any illness the appetite is the first thing to be affected. Farmers speak of a sick animal as being "off its feed." Mothers can usually tell if children are well by their eating habits. When we have been sick, often the first sign of recovery is the return of a normal appetite. All animals except us human animals stop eating when they are sick. But we often stuff and coddle the sick instead of leaving them alone to recover under nature's guidance. And our natural healing ability can often deal with our illnesses if left alone to do so!

Not surprisingly, our own natural healing efforts will often use our digestive tracts as dumping grounds, by means of belching, vomiting and salivation at one end or diarrhea, gas and increased urination at the other. Since digestive upsets of one sort or another are frequently a part of many varied kinds of illnesses, their differentiation and treatment provide a means of treating the underlying illness of which they are only part. As a single homeopathic medicine may relieve a whole collection of symptoms, by using a simple homeopathic medicine which supports, rather than opposes, these natural healing attempts of our digestive tracts, we can often cure a complex underlying illness.

For example, 13 year-old Jane S. had been vomiting for five hours before I was called to see her one December morning at 2 a.m. In addition, she had a severe headache, a constant cough, aching and weakness of her legs and aching chills—all symptoms of an influenza which was making the rounds at that time. Her vomiting came in attacks exactly one-half hour apart, and she was nauseated not only at the smell of food but from just thinking about it. This nausea, combined with the regular periodicity of her vomiting attacks and her shaking chills all are characteristic symptoms produced by *Cinchona* (or quinine). The administration of one dose of Cinchona in the 12x dilution (diluted 12 times) relieved in a few minutes not only Jane's nausea and vomiting but the headache, cough, chills and the weakness in her legs. By accepting and using Jane's digestive symptom as a key to her treatment, a whole complex disease labeled "influenza" was quickly and harmlessly relieved by *one* medicine. Therefore, in this section we are considering not solely the treatment of digestive diseases but also the use of digestive symptoms as a means of treating more complex and serious underlying illnesses. In both these areas—the relief of certain unpleasant symptoms and the use of digestive symptoms as a guide to the treatment of underlying illnesses—homeopathy has a lot to offer.

Remedies for Vomiting

Probably the most miserable GI symptom any of us can have is frequent, severe vomiting. Maybe your doctor would like to diagnose it and treat it as part of a whole picture, but you just want to get rid of it! The great homeopathic remedy for simple vomiting and nausea is Ipecac, short for *Ipecacuanha*, from the South American Tupi Indian word *ipe-caa-goéne* meaning "small plant growing by the road that makes you vomit." Its botanical name is *Cephaelis ipecacuanha*, but we will just call it Ipecac. The use of a plant which produces nausea and vomiting in the healthy for its treatment in the sick is, of course, yet another example of how homeopathy works.

The Ipecac nausea is constant and continual, accompanied by great amounts of saliva and the vomiting of large quantities of a white, shiny mucus. The nausea is not relieved by the vomiting but continues unchecked. Whatever your other symptoms or the name of your particular illness, if you have those three symptoms— excessive salivation, vomiting of profuse white mucus and constant nausea not relieved by vomiting—think of Ipecac.

It can also help many other conditions, in particular bright red bleeding from any part of the body, diarrhea from exposure to the cold, whooping cough and asthma. Six year old Henry W., the asthmatic son of an old Air Force friend, was one of my first cases, before I started my practice. He had attacks of asthma which always ended in attacks of gagging and vomiting. One dose of Ipecac 12x fixed Henry up in one day.

Another great advantage of Ipecac is that, unlike most homeopathic medicines, it is readily available from any drugstore in the form of Syrup of Ipecac, commonly used to produce vomiting in persons who have taken poison. However, for use in a homeopathic manner to relieve nausea and vomiting, this undiluted form would be incorrect. But you can easily dilute and energize it in the following manner.

Fill a small bottle with water—preferably distilled water, but tap water will do—and add to this bottle one drop of the Syrup of Ipecac, seal the bottle and strike it 15 times against the heel of your opposite hand. Pour out the contents, refill with water, reseal the bottle and strike it again 15 times against the palm of your opposite hand. By so doing you will be making a home version of the official medicines prepared by homeopathic pharmacists. Old fashioned homeopathic physicians used to prepare their medicines in this manner. Although not as desirable as medicines made by a modern homeopathic pharmacy, they may still be useful substitutes.

Some homeopathic medicines, particularly those made from botanical substances, are both safe and effective in undiluted form as tinctures. However, since some botanical tinctures such as the Foxglove (Digitalis) are violent poisons, and also since the tinctures work no differently, in my experience, than the dilutions, I recommend that you only use medicines diluted at least to the 6x level.

When the water has been poured out and refilled six times you can then use the Ipecac in that form or, best of all, repeat pouring out and refilling for a total of 12 times and use in that final form. Take a sip of this final dilution every 15 minutes until you notice relief of your symptoms. If there is no relief after three doses, discontinue the Ipecac and call your physician or, possibly, consider one of the alternative medicines for nausea and vomiting which I will mention next.

If your nausea and vomiting has not responded to Ipecac and is worse if you move in any way and better in fresh, cold air, then you might try *Tabacum*, or ordinary smoking tobacco. As any of us know who ever smoked, nausea and vomiting produced by heavy smoking is accompanied by an incredible dizziness, cold sweat and a terrible faint, sinking feeling in the pit of the stomach. Again, like Ipecac and, indeed, all homeopathic medicines, we are giving a substance to control nausea and vomiting which would produce them in healthy persons. Also, like Ipecac, you can prepare Tabacum for homeopathic use by yourself should you wish to do so, either to save money or because you don't have a local pharmacy which stocks homeopathic medicines and you can't wait to receive it from a manufacturing homeopathic pharmacist.

To prepare Tabacum for homeopathic use place a small amount of ordinary commercial tobacco (cigar tobacco would be best, as it is purest and strongest) in the bottom of a cup or heavy rolled glass. If you use cigar tobacco first shred it into small pieces. Cigarette or pipe tobacco may be used as it already comes. Cover the tobacco with pure ethyl alcohol, vodka, brandy or whisky. Since you need a doctor's prescription to purchase pure ethyl alcohol (otherwise we could make our own drinks and Uncle Sam would lose all that beautiful liquor tax money!) vodka would probably be best for you to use as it is the purest and most concentrated alcoholic drink readily available.

Let the tobacco soak in the alcohol for a few minutes and then take a spoon and mash the tobacco with it until the surrounding alcohol is colored by the tobacco. At that point, you can start a series of dilutions like the Ipecac dilution by adding one drop of the tobacco-alcohol mixture to a small bottle of water and striking the bottle against the palm of your opposite hand. When this process has been continued 12 times, as with the preceding Ipecac dilution, take a sip of the final preparation every 15 minutes for three doses. As before, if no change occurs stop at that point and consider one of the other medications for nausea and vomiting.

Another leading medicine for vomiting is the plant *Strychnos nux vomica,* from India and Ceylon. It is usually called, simply, *Nux vomica*, which is Latin for "vomiting nut." The powerful poison, Strychnine, comes from this plant. It used to be commonly used as a poison for rats and other rodents. It is not available as it once was so that you will not be able to mix your own but will have to obtain it from a homeopathic drugstore or drug supply house.

By contrast with Ipecac, the nausea of the Nux vomica patient is *relieved* by vomiting. It is immediately worse after eating and continues for an hour or so after eating and is accompanied by a heavy feeling in the stomach as if from a stone. Along with these digestive complaints goes great sensitivity and irritability to everything around—noise, lights, odors, people, criticism, coffee, tobacco smoke, alcohol, spicy food, mental overexertion, etc., etc.

A Method of Controlling Belching

Nux vomica is also a great medicine for gas from the mouth (or belching or eructations as this is called) often accompanied by a sour, or bitter taste. Although belching is considered rude in most European and American homes, in the Orient it is rude *not* to belch after a meal.

Probably the greatest homeopathic medicine for belching is ordinary charcoal, or vegetable carbon, made by burning wood in a special closed oven so that it chars instead of burning down to an ash. This is an old veterinarian's remedy for gas in animals of all types. People needing *Carbo vegetabilis* in high dilution are excessively full of gas. Their abdomen swells out like a balloon and they can belch literally for minutes on end. Lying down makes the gas worse as does eating or drinking. Belching gives immediate relief but the problem often returns.

As charcoal is used as a soil ingredient for potted plants, as well as in veterinary medicine, it is readily available to you in crude form. However, since it is not soluble in water or alcohol, it has to be prepared for homeopathic usage by grinding it with powdered milk sugar in a heavy porcelain bowl called a mortar. Then this has to be repeated in a clean mortar for each stage of dilution. You could probably use porcelain cups instead of mortars, but as they would have to be cleaned with nitric acid before they could be used again, the whole process is probably too complicated for you to undertake, particularly since homeopathic medicines are so cheap. However, in emergencies you might prepare a 6x dilution for immediate use.

The other great homeopathic medicine for belching is the Club-moss, Wolf's Foot, whose botanical name *Lycopodium clavatum* means "wolf's foot" in Latin. Persons needing this have the characteristic that their gas and belching is worse after meals. "Everything I eat turns into gas" they say. The gas is often worse at 4 in the afternoon, as are they in general. Their gas is noisy; its rumbling can be heard across the room. With it goes a painful feeling of distension and pressure around the midriff. Lycopodium persons may be gross eaters. The more they eat the more they want. They get a headache if they don't eat. And everything they eat tastes sour, leading to heartburn. If the gas pains are worse on one side of the abdomen it is usually the right side. Lycopodium is a *right-sided* medicine. Whatever the complaints, they are on the right side. Whenever you see this combination of excessive burping and rumbling gas after meals, worse at 4 p.m. and on the right side, think of Lycopodium, particularly when it is in a tense, irritable, intellectual type of person.

EffectiveTreatments for Flatus

Lycopodium is also a great medicine for gas passed by the rectum, or flatus as it is called. Judith R., one of my patients, reported that her life was made miserable by excessive, loud, smelly flatus. Such an affliction couldn't have happened to a worse person, as Judith was by nature, gentle, quiet, sensitive and self-conscious. As she was a 22 year old actress with a busy professional and social life her affliction was particularly hard to bear. I'm happy to say the Lycopodium in various dilutions over a period of months has given her great relief. She's not cured but she's a lot better!

Conditions treated by Nux vomica and Carbo vegetabilis also are accompanied by flatus, as noisy and rumbling as that of Lycopodium. The Carbo vegetabilis flatus is particularly unpleasant to smell. The Nux vomica flatus is often painful during its passage.

If your flatus smells like rotten eggs you probably need Sulfur, particularly if you have the other characteristics of Sulfur—its inner warmth, and if you desire fresh air, cold drinks and sweets, and dislike warmth, stuffy rooms or standing in one place for any length of time. Most men could do with a dose of sulfur at one time or another. Our great grandmothers used to give sulfur and molasses in the spring time. Many of the famous spas in this country as well as Europe are centered around waters high in sulfur. The mange medicines used by vets usually contain sulfur. It is a wide acting, indispensable medicine for the homeopathic physician—probably used more frequently than any of the other 2000 or more available homeopathic medicines.

Sulfur is also readily obtainable through any drugstore or chemical supply house so if you're in a hurry, you could make it up in the same manner as I suggested for Ipecac and Tabacum. Unfortunately, sulfur is insoluble in water and only slightly soluble in alcohol, so that you will have to grind it up with mild sugar to dilute it to the necessary degree for its use as a homeopathic medicine. If you're particularly sensitive to sulfur you might get a good effect by taking a glass of sulfur water at intervals. There are a number of "mineral waters"—usually meaning sulfur water—available in all parts of the country.

Another medicine for flatus is *Cinchona*, bark from the Central American tree from which quinine was first isolated (the Quichoa indian word for bark is Quina, hence the name Quinine). The person needing Cinchona is full of loud, rumbling gas which distends the abdomen like a balloon. Belching doesn't give relief but passing flatus does. With the flatus one often finds shaking chills and pains in the joints. Indeed, I have found Cinchona to be one of my most effective medications for so-called influenza attacks, associated with abdominal distension and rumbling and much smelly flatus.

Like Ipecac and some of the other medicines we have considered so far, Cinchona is readily available in drugstores in the form of quinine, or in grocery stores as "tonic" or "quinine water." Quinine is a chemical derived from cinchona bark and has a much more limited action in homeopathic usage. However, if you are bothered with flatus and have some of the other symptoms of Cinchona, quinine water may give you relief. Or, if you wish to "roll your own," since quinine is water soluble you can easily make up to a 12x dilution of it, as described before.

Remedies for Diarrhea

Along with flatus often goes diarrhea, just as nausea and vomiting accompany belching at the north end of our digestive tracts. There are so many effective homeopathic medicines for diarrhea, and so many different kinds of diarrhea, that it is hard to choose which medicines to discuss. However, regardless of cause, probably the most common form of diarrhea—as well as the most miserable—is the crampy gut ache, or "gripes" which we have all experienced at one time or another. This is the "green apple" colic we had as kids, until we learned better, where you have waves of pain in the belly making you double up, relieved after passing a watery, foul-smelling, sputtery stool, but returning soon afterwards, particularly after eating or drinking. All this adds up to a recommendation for the squirting cucumber, *Colocynthis*, and I recommend that you get some of the 12x dilution and keep it on hand for emergencies. If you need it, you need it in a hurry!

Another diarrhea medicine you should have in your home medicine kit is *Arsenicum album*, or arsenic trioxide, useful for diarrhea after eating or drinking, followed by great prostration and accompanied by severe chilliness. However, the Arsenicum diarrhea is painless. It is not preceeded by abdominal cramps made better by doubling up, and it is often burning and worse at 2 a.m. It frequently follows the intake of cold food or drinks in hot weather. Arsenicum is also one of the great homeopathic medicines for acute attacks of asthma between midnight and 2 a.m. particularly in chilly persons who can't breathe while lying flat, so that they must sit up straight.

Another great remedy for painless diarrhea is a high dilution of an old American Indian remedy, the May Apple, or *Podophyllum*. The Podophyllum diarrhea is often chronic, coming early in the morning in the form of a green, watery, profuse, foul-smelling stool and lasting till noon but followed by a normal stool in the evening. It is also helpful for diarrhea in children during teething or after eating or while being bathed or washed.

The element Sulfur is also highly indicated when chronic early morning diarrhea occurs which is also painless and foul smelling. Another medicine for early morning diarrhea is the Aloe plant from Africa and India, named *Aleo socotrina*, from the Island of Socotra in the Indian Ocean south of Arabia where it was first found. Aloe is widely used today as a basis for a facial cream for women and great claims are made for its effectiveness. Like *Colocynthis*, the Aloe diarrhea is accompanied by cutting, griping colic in the abdomen before and during a bowel movement, worse after eating or drinking and relieved after the stool, but followed by faintness often accompanied by much offensive, burning flatus, the anus burning even after the flatus has been passed.

How to Treat Hemorrhoids

Aloe is also an effective medicine for the treatment of hemorrhoids. Hemorrhoids requiring Aloe hang out of the anus like a bunch of blue grapes, and are bleeding, itching, sore, hot and tender, relieved by cold water, accompanied by an itching and burning in the anus so severe that it prevents sleep.

There are a number of outstanding homeopathic medicines for the treatment of hemorrhoids, a condition which usually responds to homeopathic treatment, often dramatically. I remember Phillip W., a 53 yr. old accountant, who had suffered from hemorrhoids for years. As Phillip stood by my desk he couldn't sit down. He told me that he had only made an appointment in order to stop his wife's nagging him to see me, and that he didn't think my "sugar pills" would do him any good. Used to such shenanigans from obstreperous male patients I went ahead with my evaluation of him anyway. He said that his hemorrhoids followed "a dose of the clap" which he had as a young man, before he was married. His gonorrhea was treated by chemical irrigation of his urethra, the standard treatment in those pre-antibiotic days. His hemorrhoids had been removed twice surgically but kept reappearing. They were large and bled easily from the touch of his clothes or a wash rag. They were worse *after* a bowel movement, lasting for hours afterwards, and felt like "a bunch of needles up my poop, Doc".

As this symptom picture was like an arrow pointing toward Nitric acid I gave him a powder of the 6x dilution of Nitric acid on his tongue and asked him to wait outside for a few minutes. When I had finished with my next patient and was showing her to my secretary's room, my hemorrhoid patient came rushing in saying "Hey Doc, I ain't got no more pain. God damn it, I hate to admit it, but I guess my old lady was right about them sugar pills!" His attacks of acute pain did not recur and over the next few months his hemorrhoids gradually shriveled down until now, so he says, there is just a "little nubbin" left, presumably of scar tissue.

The symptom of "pain like needles" is so characteristic of Nitric acid that it led me directly to that medicine. If his hemorrhoids presented the same swollen appearance of blue grapes, but instead of pricking pain like needles they had been extremely sore to the slightest touch, I would have thought of another acid for him, hydrochloric acid or in its Latin name, *Muriaticum acidum*. The Muriatic acid hemorrhoids are so tender that even the sheet is uncomfortable. They often hang out of the anus during urination.

Although both nitric and hydrochloric acids are available from many sources, they are both so poisonous and corrosive—even the fumes of nitric acid are poisonous—that I don't recommend your making your own medication from them. They are both extremely soluble in water so in emergency, if you're used to working with corrosive acids and if you use only glass bottles and stoppers in your preparation, you may get away with it but you must protect your eyes and skin carefully from any contact with the acids. Once you dilute them twelve times you could use them without any danger.

Another important hemorrhoid medicine is one familiar to all of us—the common horse chestnut (*Aesculus hippocastanum*, meaning "horse chestnut oak" in Latin and Greek) which we all collected or played with in the fall. When I was a boy we would fight with them on the ends of rawhide thongs. When the brown outer shell is removed and the remaining nut is ground in alcohol and then diluted in the usual manner it makes one of our greatest homeopathic medicines (another one from the American Indians!) The Aesculus hemorrhoids are also purplish and grape-like but their pain is of a burning quality and they rarely bleed. With them occurs a dryness of the rectum and a severe, dull ache in the lower back and hips.

Finally, two other medicines we have already considered—Nux vomica and Sulfur—are both outstanding, in high dilution, for hemorrhoids. Sulfur is particularly indicated for hemorrhoids which have been helped by other medicines but tend to recur. The hemorrhoids are painless and burn and itch but scratching makes them worse. They are worse from water and from standing but are better from cold air. In general, people requiring Sulfur are hot people who desire cold drinks and fresh air.

Nux vomica hemorrhoids often come from constipation. They itch like the Sulfur hemorrhoids but are better on cool bathing.

Effective Remedies for Constipation

Sulfur and Nux vomica are also good for constipation. You might ask how two medicines could simultaneously be good for conditions as different as constipation and diarrhea, or gas and hemorrhoids. Well, certain of the two thousand or so homeopathic medicines have very broad ranges of action so that a single medicine may help dozens of physical and/or emotional conditions. These broad-acting homeopathic medicines—there are about one hundred of them—are called *Polychrests*. The medicines emphasized in this book are largely polychrests. Nux vomica and Sulfur are two of them, particularly in their action on the entire digestive system.

The stools requiring Sulfur are large, knotty, and dry and hard as if they had been burnt. They are so painful that they cause constipation. The Nux vomica constipation is accompanied by a frequent, unsuccessful desire for a bowel movement, often in persons who have taken laxatives all their lives.

The Wild Hop, or *Bryonia alba*, is for constipation accompanied by large, dark, dry stools as if they had been burnt. In contrast with Nux vomica, the person with a Bryonia-type constipation has absolutely no desire to have a bowel movement, and will go literally weeks without one. One of my early patients—70 year old Mrs. H., a wizened-up little lady, like a dried apple—told me she had not had an 'abomination' for two weeks. It took me a minute to figure out what she meant, and when I did I feared she had an intestinal obstruction. However, she didn't seem to be in any pain, and a powder of Bryonia 12x fixed her up.

Shortly after this, another woman, Rebecca S., although this time young, plump and good natured, also had been constipated for weeks without any desire to move her bowels. Bryonia didn't help her so, after a few days I gave her a 12x dilution of the poppy, *Opium*, which gave her immediate relief.

One of the characteristics of Opium is that it often helps in cases where the apparently indicated medication has not produced relief.

This discussion of the homeopathic treatment of illnesses of the digestive tract has been necessarily sketchy. Only a few of the most common and most effective medicines for each complaint and only a few of the most common digestive troubles have been considered. Nevertheless, however sketchy, this chapter should have introduced you to the ever-fascinating subject of homeopathic treatment. You may be assured that whatever your complaint—digestive or otherwise—homeopathic treatment will probably have something to offer.

2

Homeopathic Medicines for a Healthy Heart

As we all must be aware, coronary heart disease is the greatest killer of men over 40 in this country and, indeed, in most wealthy, industrialized countries. Like a thief in the night it strikes suddenly—usually without warning—killing one half of its victims within the first few days.

Human Productivity and Heart Health

Doubly tragic is that heart disease *selects* its victims from among the leaders of our society—men of above average physical strength (many are ex-athletes) as well as intelligence and will to succeed. The hard-driving, competitive, business executive or professional man is a typical victim. Statistically, coronary heart disease is most common among physically inactive, overweight, and emotionally tense persons with high blood pressure, a high level of fats in the blood, a family tendency to heart disease, responsible occupations, and an excessive intake of animal fats in their diet.

Coronary heart disease is the most dramatic type of heart disease. It takes its name from the coronary artery which like a crown (Latin *Corona*) surrounds the upper part of the heart, both front and back, sending feeding arteries to the muscles controlling its four walled chambers.

Differences Between Heart Spasms and Heart Infarctions

When the coronary arteries momentarily constrict—particularly if they are partially plugged by fat—a severe crushing pain is felt in the heart. This is generally called a coronary spasm, or more technically, angina pectoris. These attacks are often brought on by eating, emotional stress or by exertion, particularly walking in a cold wind. The famous London surgeon, John Hunter, who suffered from coronary heart disease, said "My life is in the hands of any rascal who chooses to annoy and tease me."

Although coronary spasms are a sign that something is wrong with the heart they are not necessarily fatal. Some persons may live with them for many years.

By contrast, if a branch of the coronary artery is closed permanently, either by filling gradually with fatty deposits, (like the water pipes in an old house) or suddenly by a blood clot carried from elsewhere in the body, the section of heart muscle supplied by that branch of the coronary artery will die, becoming replaced by scar tissue (called an infarct).

Such an event is truly catastrophic. The pain is so severe it blots out all other awareness, so that one becomes, simply, pure pain. If a major area of the heart is affected, death may be immediate. If a relatively minor area is affected, recovery although slow, is possible, leaving the owner of the heart a permanent cripple.

Although coronary artery disease is the most serious of heart diseases, unfortunately it is not the only cause. There are many others, such as rheumatic fever, infections, inheritance, high blood pressure, endocrine gland disorders (as accompanies an underactive thyroid) and injuries. Even syphillis, tuberculosis and trichinosis from spoiled pork may affect the heart.

How to Treat Heart Attacks

In spite of these many causes of heart disease, homeopathy can treat them all by means of a person's symptoms without tailoring the treatment toward one diagnosis or another. For example, many years ago I was called to the hotel room of Mr. Paul R. That afternoon he had suffered a severe, crushing chest pain after a luncheon at his hotel with some business associates. The hotel physician found definite electrocardiographic evidence of a coronary artery event.

On examining him I found an extremely agitated, frightened man of about 45 in intense pain, bathed in cold perspiration, with a weak, thready pulse, complaining of a crushing pain over his breast-bone and a feeling as if his chest were squeezed in a wire cage. Since all this was a classic picture of conditions produced by the great night blooming flower of our southwestern desert, *Cactus Grandiflorus*, I immediately placed a 12x dilution of Cactus on his tongue. Mr. R. experienced almost immediate relief of the pain, continuing through the night. Incidently, Cactus also relieved his fear of death, as well as his anger and irritability. (An old nurse told me she hated working in a cardiac ward because the patients were so cantankerous). Although severely shaken by his heart attack, Mr. R. remained comfortable during his convalescence. As usual, I put him on a diet low in animal fats, as follows:

Recommendations

1. *EGGS*

   Eat as many egg whites as you wish.

2. *DAIRY FOODS*

   Eat only buttermilk, skim milk, sherbet, and fat-free cottage or pot cheese.

3. *MEATS*

   Chicken, turkey and veal in 4 oz. portions may be eaten three times per week. In addition, eat at least five meals a week of finned fish, such as tuna, salmon, halibut etc. Eat shellfish such as shrimp, crab, lobster, oyster and clams etc., not more than once in two weeks.

Prohibitions

Eat no more than four egg yolks a week.

Eat no other cheeses than cottage, pot or farmer cheese and eat no cream, butter, ice cream or whole milk.

Eat no more than 15 oz. (an adult male's palm is about 4 oz.) a week of beef, pork, lamb, or delicatessen meats, such as salami, liverwurst, bologna, etc. Use no lard, suet or chicken fat in cooking.

Recommendations	Prohibitions

4. *FRUITS AND
   VEGETABLES*

You may eat any fruits, vegetables, nuts and grains you wish in any amount save for cashews, coconut and chocolate. A substitute for chocolate is CAROB, available as a powder or confection at health food stores. Eat only margarines that list liquid vegetable oil as their primary ingredient.

Eat no cashews, chocolate, or coconut in any form. Avoid products containing shortening, vegetable fat, or hydrogenated vegetable oil. Use only vegetable oil in cooking

5. *BREADS AND PASTRIES*

You may eat low fat content breads and pastries such as bread, rolls, biscuits, angel food cake, sponge cake, almond macaroons, or honey cake; eat high fat content pastries such as pies, or cookies if they contain only natural, unaltered vegetable oils.

Please eat no pies, cookies, cakes or pastries, doughnuts, muffins or crackers prepared with coconut oil, lard, butter, crisco or hydrogenated vegetable oils.

This diet helps prevent further heart attacks.

Although many homeopathic medicines for heart trouble come from plants and minerals also, it is interesting that many are made from snake and insect products. In nature these usually act by destruction of elements in the blood stream, therefore their usefulness for heart conditions. They are best used in dilutions greater than the 12th decimal (12x).

Chief among the snake medicines for heart trouble is a cobra venom, *Naja Naja Naja*. As in cases requiring *Cactus grandiflorus*, persons needing high dilutions of Naja are often suicidal, frequently from brooding over imaginary troubles. There is a severe stitching pain in the region of the heart accompanied by a pulse irregular in strength but not in beat. There is a feeling of weakness in the heart, and, indeed, the particular area of action of this medicine is in hearts weakened by previous attacts of acute inflammation or from chronic cardiac enlargement due to imperfect heart valves. The violent, cramping pain in the heart extends to the left shoulder and neck or to the left shoulder blade. There is an excited, tremendous heaving action of the heart; clearly seen in the left breast. Frequently the heart is enlarged, from valvular damage, high blood pressure or other causes. The pain is worse lying on the left side and better in the open air. Homeopathic physicians treat persons with these symptoms with high dilutions of Naja—dilutions so high that no snake venom is still present, only it's energy effect.

By contrast with Naja, a person suffering from a condition requiring a high dilution of rattlesnake venom, *Crotalus Horridus*, is worse lying on the *right* side. He also has a weakness of the heart and experiences a strange feeling "as if the heart turns over in the chest." Like the dark, foul pits where rattlesnakes dwell there is a putridity, a darkness and malignancy about the symptoms of someone requiring this snake venom. There are dark hemorrhages. The parts affected have a dusky, bluish look. The face is dark, the fingernails blue—all classic signs of a lack of oxygen due to cardiac impairment. Even the dreams are horrible, often of death and the dead. Anyone who has ever seen a case of rattlesnake bite will recognize the putridity and the purplish color of the wound. Cardiac patients with these symptoms may benefit from *Crotalus Horridus* in high dilutions (above the 30th decimal).

Many cardiac patients suffer pains in the left arm. Neurologically, both the heart and the left arm are supplied by associated nerves so that what affects one may affect the other by referred pain, just as the area under the right shoulder blade may develop pain in the presence of gall bladder trouble because both areas are supplied by the same nerve section.

Another high dilution of venom, this time from an insect—the black widow spider—is outstanding for treatment of this radiation of heart pain into the left arm. The scientific name of this spider is *Latrodectus mactans*. The heart pain is violent, radiating to both shoulders, in particular the left. The patient gasps with pain, fearing to lose breath and die. The pulse is quick and thready. Any exertion makes the patient worse. Homeopathic physicians relieve these symptoms with *Lactrodectus mactans* in 12x dilutions.

Finally, another poisonous substance good for heart trouble—this time a plant—is *Tabacum* (from the Taino word Tabaco, meaning a rolled leaf of tobacco). Although many think of tobacco as a pleasant tranquilizer, nicotine (the chief alkaloid in tobacco) is a violent poison—nicotine from half a cigar is enough to kill an adult human if injected into the blood stream. The use of *Tabacum* in heart disease follows, of course, the homeopathic premise, that what causes symptoms in healthy people may relieve them in the sick.

As frequently emphasized throughout this book, homeopathic medicines are diluted to such a degree that none of the original substance is left, only its energy effect. Therefore, they are safe and non-toxic—even though their starting medicines may be snake venoms, poisonous herbs like strychnine or poisonous chemicals like Mercury.

As any smoker knows, before becoming "hooked," our initial reactions to tobacco smoking are paroxysms of dizziness, weakness, seasickness, vomiting, and chilliness with a cold sweat, often accompanied by headaches, diarrhea and palpitations of the heart. In the face of such a profound reaction, why any of us go on and acquire the nicotine habit shows how much we are bound by the opinion of others.

Some years ago my patient Mr. Kenneth X., a 40-year old stockbroker, suffered a heart attack accompanied by nausea, chilliness, weakness, and other symptoms identical to that of tobacco poisoning. Tabaccum in the 12x homeopathic potency gave Mr. X. quick relief. As both the heart and the stomach are supplied by branches of the same nerve—the *Vagus* (from the Latin *Vagus*, meaning "wandering" hence our word vagabond)—we can easily understand such an association between heart and stomach troubles.

In addition to its general nicotine-like poisoning symptoms, certain symptoms specifically related to heart attacks may respond to Tabaccum. In particular, one is the *twisting* pain about the heart, the very twisty pain from which angina pectoris is named. Unlike other heart medicine like cobra and rattlesnake venom—hard to get in the local supermarket—Tabaccum is only as far away as the nearest store, so you can readily prepare you own Tabaccum in *homeopathic* form to the 12x dilution should you care to do so.

Before leaving our discussion of medicine for heart attacks we should consider the innocuous sounding pinkroot, *Spigelia Marilandica.* Effects of this plant on humans includes violent, audible palpitations of the heart and severe, shocking or compressive pains. With this comes a great sensitivity to touch of any part of the body. The heart pains are worse from motion and cold, wet weather. When these symptoms are present, Spigelia in the 6x or 12x dilution is often helpful.

Remedies for Heart Failure

Unfortunately, heart attacks are only one of the many types of heart disease to which we humans are subject. Heart enlargement is one of the most serious and chronic forms of heart trouble. The enlargement may be due to weakness of the valves or of the wall of the heart, an abnormal secretion of hormones, a direct infection, or it may be secondary to the destruction and scarring of the heart from a heart attack.

Whatever the initial cause, many pathological changes soon follow.

Because the heart has become inefficient as a pump, poorly oxygenated blood piles up in the lungs and in the veins of the upper extremities and the face. This makes for shortness of breath on exertion and bluish tinged fingernails and lips. Also, fluid may collect in the lungs, producing asthmatic wheezing, worse on lying flat, and gurgles and crackling noises readily heard with a stethoscope and often apparent to an observer on the other side of the room. As the disease progresses the liver enlarges, producing an extended, painful fluid-filled abdomen, and the kidneys degenerate, producing swollen, fluid-filled ankles and feet.

One of the best medicines for this truly pitiable group of symptoms is ordinary vegetable charcoal—the kind we're used to feeding pets when they are too gassy (or taking ourselves, for the same reason). When prepared in homeopathic potency, and tested on healthy humans, plain everyday charcoal develops many of the classic symptoms of heart enlargement and failure. The face is pale, pinched, sweaty and cold. The skin is blue and the extremities cold, so cold they interfere with sleep. There is a constant desire to be fanned, a weakness of memory and slowness of thought. And, of course, there is excessive flatulence, often so distending the abdomen as to make any position uncomfortable. When these symptoms are present, *Carbo vegetabilis* in the 6x or 12x potency should help. If you wish, by following the directions in Chapter 1 on intestinal diseases, you can prepare your own.

Another gassy medicine I have found of particular value in heart failure is *Lycopodium clavatum*, a common, yellow mold. A dilution of 12x soon relieved Mrs. Z., a little old lady of 85, and a patient of mine, who had developed severe swelling of her ankles following a series of heart attacks. This was early in my professional life and I was surprised to see Lycopodium work out from her symptoms as the most likely medicine. Since then I consider Lycopodium first for swollen ankles from any cause.

Another great medicine for cardiac failure is *Apis mellifica*, made from the crushed body of the honeybee. This unusual medicine is good for swelling of the feet and hands, accompained by swelling under the eyes. There is often urinary frequency with great irritation of the urinary apparatus, so it is hard to hold the urine even for a moment, and the urine scalds the parts over which it passes. Also, there is great sensitivity to heat and stuffy rooms. As before, the 6x or 12x dilution is often useful for persons with these conditions. If you can catch a Queen bee you can prepare your own medicine, but it must be a queen, not an ordinary bee.

Apis mellifica is often good for persons made ill by jealously, like the Queen bee who likes to have all the men to herself.

If the heart failure has resulted from organic heart disease, *Arsenicum iodatum*, arsenic iodide, in a small dilution (the 12x) is often useful. The pulse is rapid and irritable and the heart action weak. Usually these patients are chilly and short of breath and often have a hacking cough. They are worse in dry, cold or windy weather or on exertion and, like Apis, are better in the open air.

Another useful medicine in a small dilution (the 6x or 12x) for heart failure from any cause is the South African arrow poison, *Strophanthus hispidus*. Like Arsenicum iodatum ,it is used when the pulse is small, frequent and irregular and the breath is short. However, *Strophanthus* often has a burning in the throat and stomach, with nausea and vomiting. There is a feeling of lively action in the heart. The forearms and fingers may feel heavy and there may be twitching and increased secretions from all parts of the body.

The plant *Strophanthus*,contains a number of substances called glycosides, consisting of a molecule of sugar connected to another substance called a "genin" or "aglucone." Since these glycosides act on the heart they are called cardiac glycosides. A number of plants contain cardiac glycosides.

Chief among these plants is the Foxglove, or *Digitalis purpurea*, introduced into medicine by William Withering of England in 1773. Actually, Withering didn't introduce it. He found out about it from a local woman who had inherited it as a family recipe for curing the "dropsy," (swelling of the extremities). On checking over her recipe, which contained many herbs, Withering found the Foxglove to be the active ingredient.

Since then Foxglove has been a mainstay for physicians in their treatment of cardiac problems. It has been shown to contain a number of cardiac glycosides, chiefly digitoxin, gitalin and gitoxin. Most of us are familiar with these as products used by the average physician (along with the dried Digitalis leaf).

In homeopathic use, *Digitalis purpurea* is given for the symptoms it may produce in healthy volunteers. These symptoms provide uses for digitalis which often differ from those of the average physician. For instance, as a result of heart damage the beat regulation is often interfered with so that the heart beats rapidly and irregularly (fibrillates). Digitalis is used by non-homeopathic physicians to *reduce* this heart beat to a more normal level. However, the homeopathic physician will give digitalis to a person with an abnormally *slow* pulse rate, since that is the action of digitalis on healthy persons.

This may seem puzzling, and at first sight the common method of using digitalis for rapid hearts seems to make more sense. However, the significant difference is that in non-homeopathic use, digitalis helps reduce the rapid heart beat but does not remove it, so that the patient must continue taking the digitalis each day, sometimes for a lifetime. In homeopathic use, however, digitalis would not be used for a rapid heart beat. One of our other medicines such as Pinkroot (*Spigelia*), or Deadly Nightshade (*belladonna*), would be used. These might slow the heart and also prevent the fibrillation from returning, so that after they are discontinued their effect would continue.

Thus, in homeopathic usage, *Digitalis purpurea* would be used for persons with *slow*, not *rapid*, heart beats. Among patients with cardiac failure it is of particular value in hearts weak from causes other than valvular complications. A retired naval officer, Malcolm J., suffered from faintness and sinking at the stomach with exhaustion and extreme prostration and a feeling as if he were dying. His chest was so weak that talking was difficult. His skin was pale and bluish with distended veins on the lids, ears, lips and tongue; his fingers went to sleep easily. Two doses of digitalis in the 12x dilution relieved his symptoms in two days. Digitalis is of particular value in swelling after scarlet fever, or Bright's Disease, with suppression of the urine.

Another medicine important in cardiac dropsy is Canadian Hemp, *Apocynum Cannabinum*. It also contains a cardiac glycoside, cymarin, closely related to strophanin, the glycoside of Strophanthus.

This medicine is of value in dropsy following infections such as typhus or typhoid fever or scarlatine, or after cirrhosis of the liver or overdosing with quinine. These patients, although thirsty, find that water disagrees with them, sometimes producing nausea and even vomiting. Most of these persons do not have organic heart disease. For instance, Mrs. Ruth N., a retired school teacher, had suffered for many years from symptoms like the foregoing, but all tests for organic heart disease were negative. In spite of the long duration of her illness, two doses of Apocynum 6x dilution, at intervals of 12 hours between the two doses, relieved her symptoms within 12 hours.

Since Canadian Hemp grows commonly in country places, you can readily prepare a 6x or 12x dilution of the tincture, should you care to do so.

3

How to Treat External Ailments with Homeopathic Medicines

Here we will consider the treatment of all those external illnesses—such as cuts, bruises, fractures, sprains, etc.—which start happening to most of us as soon as we're born.

Earlier medical textbooks spoke of internal medicine for illnesses that arise from within and external medicine dealing with illnesses arising from external causes. Internal medicine was the province of the physician; external medicine of the surgeon. As physicians and surgeons became more closely allied (three hundred years ago surgeons were a different profession entirely) the difference between these two natural divisions in medicine tended to blur, particularly with the development of the so-called medical specialties (actually predominantly surgical) from their beginning. Only in very recent years has internal medicine developed specialities like cardiology or endocrinology. The early specialties—such as eye, obstetrics and gynecology, ear, nose and throat, etc.—were all surgical.

Remarkable Results of Homeopathic Remedies
for Common Injuries

Nowadays external medicine would be called traumatic medicine. Although homeopathy is strictly a medical specialty, it has numerous medicines of value in treating accidents and injuries of many types. Unless otherwise indicated, these medicines are to be taken by mouth.

Chief among them is the herb Leopard's Bane, or *Arnica Montana*. If you find it in your garden, or get the dried plant from an herbalist, you can prepare your own 6x or 12x dilution from the alcoholic tincture of the plant, as described earlier in Chapter 1 on intestinal problems. I have used this routinely for patients before and after operations, or following injuries of any type, and its action is so remarkable that even after 20 years of practice I am still amazed by it. Sometimes I think if homeopathy had done nothing but introduce this medicine into general use, it would have justified its existence. In my opinion, every family should have Arnica available in a home kit, and every physician should be aware of its use and *use* it. Arnica is particularly valuable after bruises and the effects of falls, or stiffness from long riding, and also for excessive physical fatigue. It's even good as a foot bath, for tired feet, by placing a few drops in the water. It's particularly good before delivery as it make childbirth quicker and more comfortable. Through the years I must have used it in hundreds of women before childbirth and the results are consistently marvelous. Often their obstetricians will comment on the lack of complication and their speedy recovery.

Treating Wounds and Cuts

Everything on which the Arnica patient sits seems too hard. There is a sore, lame, bruised feeling throughout the body as if beaten. Arnica is great for poorly healed wounds or for persons who have not felt well since an operation or accident. The length of time since the injury appears not to matter.

I remember a friend of mine, Herbert N., who had suffered severe back pains since a diving accident 20 years before. One dose of

Arnica 6x fixed him up in two days. After Jessica W. a secretary in her middle thirties suffered a "whiplash" injury in an automobile accident she developed a host of complex troubles both physical and psychological. In addition to serious neck pains and gastric problems, she was weepy, suspicious, and emotionally and mentally disoriented. Arnica 12x in a series of doses over a period of months gradually relieved her symptom complex.

How to Treat Bruises

Another great remedy for bruises and cuts is the common field daisy, *Bellis perennis.* As this is readily available in the spring and summer you can prepare your own medicine. Just as this is so tough that it pops up again if you walk on it, so patients with bruises and cuts will "pop up" again after a bit of *Bellis perennis* in homeopathic potency. (I find the 6x particularly useful). *Bellis perennis* is also good for deep traumatic or infected wounds, as well as general fatigue and tiredness.

The great medicine for wounds of all types is the common marigold, *Calendula officinalis,* also readily available to you for home preparation. Many persons use it as a salve or ointment. It is particularly useful for *painful* wounds, if they are open, torn, cut, lacerated, ragged or oozing pus. Also, in hemorrhages from scalp wounds or after drawing teeth it is useful in oral form. And, taken by mouth it also helps prevent wound infections and disfiguring scars. It is helpful in nerve tumors or inflammation following an injury, and also in persons exhausted from blood loss and excessive pain. Ruptured muscles and tendons or tears during childbirth or wounds that penetrate joints producing loss of joint fluid also frequently respond to Calendula.

Witch hazel (*Hamamelis Virginica*), again readily available to you for home preparation, is the grand old lotion of athletic trainers and gyms. It's useful for bruises and sprains like Arnica, and , like Arnica, also for incised, lacerated or contused wounds or injuries from falls or for bleeding from any cause particularly from the uterus after riding over rough roads. It's also great for inflammation of the white of your eyes (conjunctivitis), from injury, or maybe from rubbing them too hard when you get a cinder in your eye.

In fact, Hamamelis and Arnica are so much alike that they can be used almost interchangeable—I usually start first with Arnica, but you could start with Hamamelis. In a sense Hamamelis is better because most drugstores carry the tincture in rubbing alcohol. Unfortunately the rubbing alcohol is poisonous, so you can't drink that, but must rub it on. If you can get the pure alcoholic tincture, put a drop in a glass of water and knock it against the heel of your hand fifteen times. Empty the glass quickly, so a little clings to the inside, and refill with water. Repeat the whole process six times and you have about a 6x (or 6 decimal) dilution, which you can then sip directly from the glass. In this form, one sip is equal to one pinch of powdered medicine, and should be repeated only a few times in accordance with the earlier instruction.

We have all banged our toes or shins against things around the house. As kids we were frequently kicked in the shins playing games. These bone bruises can go very deep and hurt for a long time afterwards. I remember the father of one of my boyhood friends who had been soccer champion of England as a young man. His shins were still covered with bruises 20 years later.

The herb Rue (*Ruta graveolens*) is specific for bone bruises, or injuries of the tissues surrounding the bone (periosteum) as well as for sprains and dislocations. William W., a man of 42, came to me because of complaints following his first mountain climbing trip of the season. He had a bruised lame feeling all over, with pain in parts of the body on which he lay, along with a deep pain in the bones, which was made better by walking around. A 12x dilution of Rue fixed him up in 12 hours. Rue is also good for complaints from overexertion, even of the eye.

How to Treat Punctured Wounds

Finally, if parts rich in nerves are injured, or for any punctured wound like those from stepping on a nail, take St. John's Wort (*Hypericum perforatum*), or Marsh Tea (*Ledum palustre*). Ledum is also good for animal bites and insect stings, particularly from mosquitos.

A Remedy for Mosquito Bites and Cuts

Incidentally, speaking of mosquitos, the Delphinium or Stavesacre plant, *Staphisagria*, according to folk legend helps keep mosquitos away. Dr. J., one of my colleagues, uses it in the 12x dilution for a number of his patients and says it helps. For instance, the T. family of five, all sensitive to mosquitos, noticed relief in one day. Staphisagria is also good for injuries from sharp-cutting instruments, as after surgical operations. It has a stinging, smarting pain like the cutting of a knife. Staphisagria patients are extremely sensitive, full of anger, indignation, grief and mortification.

To return to Hypericum, in addition to crushed wounds (as fingertips), it is also good for mechanical injuries to the spinal cord resulting in concussion or headaches, or for bad falls on the back, or pain after falling on the coccyx. As you may remember, the coccyx is the little "monkey's tail" bone on the end of the spine. It's only purpose seems to be to make trouble for women, whose pelvic bones are more open than in men so that the coccyx is more easily injured. I have had dozens of women compain to me of troubles following falls on the coccyx; I can't remember a single man doing so. As nerves from the coccyx go to the pelvic organs, women often have menstrual or ovarian problems following injuries to the coccyx. The coccyx is often injured in childbirth.

Hypericum 12x can usually help these unfortunate ladies. Also, massage or manipulation of the coccyx can often help.

Hypericum is also good for the nervous depression which often follows wounds or surgical operations. It removes the bad effects of shock or fright. Also, the older books say it is good for the bad effects of mesmerism (hypnotism)!

Just to finish off *Ledum palustre*. In addition to punctured wounds and bites, Ledum 12x dilution usually gives immediate relief for bruising injuries to the eyes and eyelids, particularly if there is much bleeding under the skin. In other words, it's good for black eyes, particularly the ripe, purple ones! Along the same line, it is good for "black and blue" discolorations that stay a long time after injuries, particularly if they become green.

Ledum is good for sprains, in people with weak ankles and feet, who are always spraining them. The relief is usually immediate.

The Importance of Subjective Symptoms

How to tell Ledum, Hypericum and Staphisagria patients apart, since they're all good for puncture injuries? Well, patients needing Ledum are strange. They feel chilly all the time, and their wounded parts are chilly to the touch, but their pains are better from cold (even icy) water, or cool air, and they are worse from warm covers or air. Mrs. Henry B., a 32-year old housewife presented this typical Ledum picture and responded well to the 6x dilution. Mrs. James D., on the other hand, a typical patient needing Hypericum presented no such paradoxical picture. She was worse from the cold, the damp, from fog and from changing weather, and was helped by Hypericum 12x. Both ladies were hypersensitive to any jar or motion, as are most Hypericum and Ledum patients. Like Hypericum, Staphisagria patients are worse from cold, (but from *cold drinks*, not primarily from cold), damp and fog, and unlike Ledum, are better with warmth. Staphisagria patients in contrast to Ledum patients are extremely sensitive to the least *touch* on the affected parts. Hypericum patients also have this sensitivity.

This little differentiation between the homeopathic use of Hypericum, Ledum and Staphisagria illustrates the richness of the homeopathic method of therapy. Because the medicines are first tested in great detail on healthy persons, a whole, complex understanding of their action is obtained. Each medicine becomes a personality, with its own subtle physical, emotional and mental sphere of action. The inclusion of subjective (or inner) as well as the objective (or outer) reaction of the test subjects makes this differentiation possible.

Unusual Remedies for Insect Bites

In our crowded world bites and stings of various kinds are always with us. We already considered Staphisagria and Ledum for mosquito bites. Ledum is good for the effects of insect, bee and animal poisons in general. For ant stings a homeopathic preparation of *Formica rufa* (the ant) is often helpful. Bee stings often respond to *Apis mellifica*, the Queen bee; wasp stings to *Vespa crabro*, the wasp; and spider stings to *Tarentula cubensis*, the tarantula spider. All the other stinging insects are either available in homeopathic potency, or for a modest fee can be specially made up by a homeopathic pharmacy such as Ehrhart & Kart in Chicago. So many of my patients, largely women, were allergic to flea bites that I obtained a few different dilutions of *Pulex irritans*, the common flea, for my use. Its done yeoman's service. Mrs. Joanne F., a woman in her forties, in addition to swollen ankles and legs from just one flea bite, would get sick all over with headaches, nausea and general "all-goneness." One summer she rented a house in the country which was so saturated with fleas that they rose like a cloud above the living room rug. Thanks to the administration of Pulex 6x, and the use of some insecticide, her summer was saved from catastrophe. Unfortunately for them, patients with this flea sensitivity appear to have great "flea appeal." They can be with a crowd of people and if there's one flea in a room it ends up on them. As I think about it, I have never known a man to have this type of reaction, only women. Ticks can also be a problem. Nancy E., a girl of 8, had a bald spot on her head for 2 years following a tick bite, a present from their dog. Nancy brought in a tick for me from the same dog. This tick, made into a 12x dilution, removed the bald spot within one month. All these insect remedies you can prepare yourself if you can catch a suitable insect.

Other than this use of the specific insect for treatment of the effects of its bite, in homeopathic practice there are a number of medicines for the effects of bites in general. The stinging nettle, *Urtica urens*, is helpful in bee stings. A drop of Arnica tincture applied to a wasp sting usually cures it at once. When stings become inflamed and infected—as gnat bites will often become —Cantharis is of value.

Treatment of Sprains and Strains

Sprains and strains are a frequent problem, particularly in older people whose coordination and flexibility are poor. For fresh sprains the first medicine to start with is our old friend *Arnica montana*. This can be used both internally and externally by taking a pinch on the tongue and at the same time soaking the injured part in hot water in which a few drops of the alcoholic tincture of arnica were placed. If this doesn't give relief in 48 hours then repeat both the internal and external medication using *Bellis perennis* in place of the Arnica.

Older sprains often call for other medicines. If the sprain is worse after rest and cold or damp, and better after exercise or warmth or dryness, try a 12x dilution of poison ivy, or *Rhus toxicodendron*. If it is worse from cold and damp and better from warmth and dryness but *not* relieved by exercise, try a 12x dilution of the oyster shell—*Calcarea ostrearum*.

A medicine related to *Rhus toxicodendron* for sprains is *Ruta graveolens* (Rue). Like Rhus tox it is worse from the damp and cold and lying or sitting, and better from dry, warmth and motion (although it is better lying on the back). However, it is a deeper acting medicine than Rhus tox. Think of Ruta when the picture appears to be Rhus tox but the pain extends deep into the bones and along the lining of the bones (called the periosteum). Also, with Ruta the entire body may feel bruised and painful so the patient turns and changes position frequently. You can readily prepare Ruta from your own garden.

Strains and sprains are nature's way of protecting us from fractures, by letting a joint bend rather than allowing a bone to break. However, fractures do occur and may benefit from homeopathic treatment.

Of course, no medication can make a bone set itself. If bones are out of place they must be brought into proper alignment before they can knit. Proper alignment is brought about by "reducing" the fracture, that is, moving the bones either directly by hand or indirectly by means of traction devices. Most fractures can be set without operating, called "closed reduction." Sometimes the fracture must be exposed by surgery, known as "open" reduction. This is necessary where the fracture is too complex for union by simple closed reduction, as in what is called a "spiral" fracture of the tibia, or bone of the lower leg. A spiral fracture, as the name implies, goes in an "S" form up and down the shaft of the long bone. Spiral fractures of the leg frequently occur from sking accidents. The particles of bone often must be held together with a plate for the fracture to heal.

Treatment of Fractures

Even before the bone has been set, when the fracture has first been diagnosed, an ancient folk herb called, appropriately "bone set," often helps to relieve the pain of the fracture. Its scientific name is *Symphytum officinalis*, and is probably another herb from your garden. It speeds the union of fractured bones and is specific for the peculiar kind of pricking pain or for the pain along the shaft of broken bones (the periosteum) which often follows fractures. In addition it is helpful for pains from old wounds in the periosteum or cartilage which did not involve an actual fracture.

Symphytum is also helpful for pain of the eyeball following bruises or blows.

If the fractured bones are much injured or bruised, our old friend *Ruta graveolens* is helpful. As you may remember, with Ruta there is an aching, bruised feeling over the entire body. Twenty-two year old Hank Z., a hippie from San Francisco, was thrown from his motorcycle and broke a leg. Because he was dragged by his motorcycle after he was thrown, the leg bone was bruised as was his whole body. Ruta 12x gave him much relief within a few hours.

Once the fracture has been set, another medicine which speeds healing is *Calcarea phosphoricum* or Calcium phosphate. This is, as you know, one of the most common components of bones. It is of particular value in conditions of non-union of the bones, and also, in children, where the bones in the head are too thin and brittle, where the child has delayed and complicated teething, or when the spaces between the cranial bones of infants (called fontanelles and sutures) remain open too long, or close and then re-open.

The Many Helpful Remedies for Burns

Burns are another common acute injury we have all suffered at one time or another. Homeopathic treatment has a number of internal and external methods of treating them. For mild burns that don't form blisters, a tincture of the common nettle, *Urtica urens*, in water applied as a lotion on wet rags is often effective. If the burn forms blisters a lotion of witch hazel, *Hamamelis virginica*, may be used in the same manner.

One of my most effective medicines for superficial burns is everyday Cayenne pepper, *Capsicum annuum.* Like nettles, and Witch Hazel, red pepper is readily available for your own home preparation should you wish. Anyone who has taken too much red pepper knows how similar are its hot effects to the feeling of a burn. Jonathan D., a 6-year old boy, burned himself on the stove. Capsicum ointment in the 6x dilution gave him immediate relief.

If the burn has extended far enough into the skin to form blisters, then a tincture of Spanish fly, *Cantharides*, should be applied locally and also, in higher dilution, by mouth. If the blisters are deep enough to destroy the skin, so that open, running ulcers form, then potassium bichromate (*Kali bichromicum*) may be of value. If the burns become infected, then Sulphuret of Lime, (*Hepar sulphuris*) is often useful.

An unusual condition, happily, for most of us are X-ray burns. They often respond to the homeopathic medicine, X-ray, made, interestingly enough, by exposing milk sugar to X-rays and using that as a medicine in the 6x or 12x dilution.

Other ways we suffer injuries are from onslaughts from our surroundings—as too much sun, water, food—or from poisons such as contaminated food. Homeopathy also has medicines for these conditions.

How to Treat Sunstroke

For the immediate effects of sunstroke, nitroglycerine (*Glonoine*) in 6x or 12x dilution is often effective. In sunstroke the head feels enormous, as if the skull were too small for the brain, often accompanied by a pulsating, throbbing headache which is worse at every pulsation of the blood or at every jar and step. Even a brief walk in the sun, exposure to the heat of a fire, or working under hot, bright lights can affect sensitive persons badly.

Once it starts, the headache may continue even in the shade but coincides with the circuit of the sun, increasing and decreasing as the sun rises, reaches its zenith, and then sets. The crown of the head, and spine, feel hot. Zygmont R., a 40-year old teacher had headaches of this type and received help from Glonoine 6x in 10 minutes.

Sometimes the sunstroke may lead to the rupture of an artery in the brain, producing a "stroke" or, technically, a cerebrovascular accident or "CVA". Glonoine may also help persons with this condition.

If a person with sunstroke feels dull and stupid and notices an outward pressing of the head combined with great physical restlessness, anxiety and fear of death, the Monkshood, *Aconitum napellus*, may help. The skin is dry and hot, the face red, or alternately red and pale, and there is a great burning thirst for large amounts of cold water.

If dizziness is present, with staggering on trying to move and a band-like pain around the head, over the eyes, a 6x dilution of the Yellow Jasmine, *Gelsemium sempervirens*, may be helpful. There is often a general depression, with weakness and trembling and a desire to be let alone, and a confusion and lack of muscular coordination so that the muscles refuse to obey the will.

How to Treat Seasickness

Motion sickness is another common illness of our environment—funny to everyone but the sufferer, who is certain death is near. It's impact is so severe that some people will become frightened *before* the voyage starts. For them a high dilution of the Monkshood, *Aconitum napellus*, may help. The Aconitum fear is intense, making life miserable, and is accompanied by a restless tossing about. Janice R. was a *nonfearing* traveler, but she knew from previous bitter experience that her nausea and vomiting were usually accompanied by dizziness and an empty feeling in the head. A 12x dilution of the herb *Cocculus Indicus*, a few days before leaving, and a few times a day during the trip, gave her relief. Janice was nauseated even by *looking* at a boat in motion. She also usually suffered a loss of appetite, a metallic taste and a headache in the back of the head with the nausea and vomiting, combined with a tiredness of the whole body so extreme that it required all her energy to stand firmly or to speak or even to move the bowels.Thus, constipation while traveling is often an indication for Cocculus. Monkshood, Cocculus and Jasmine are readily available from your gardens, so should you wish to you can prepare them yourselves according to the earlier direction.

If the nausea and vomiting are accompanied by profound prostration and cold sweat, ordinary tobacco, *Tabacum officinalis*, often dramatically and promptly relieves the symptoms. You can of course prepare your own medicine if you wish as already described in previous chapters. Smokers will recognize in this group of symptoms their first experiments with tobacco. That any of us go on to become chronic smokers, after such a first reaction, bespeaks the social pressures which surround us all.

4

Helping Psychological Illnesses the Homeopathic Way

The Psychoneurotic Basis of Many Illnesses

According to conservative estimates, at least one-third of all the patients in doctors' offices, nursing homes and hospitals in this country have some type of psychoneurotic disease. Of course this kind of judgment is extremely difficult to make since no accepted definition of "psychoneurotic disease" has ever been produced. There is a general agreement as to what constitutes insanity, or the true psychoses, the most serious form of psychological illness. By contrast, authorities differ widely among themselves as to what is and is not psychoneurotic, particularly since the authorities argue from entirely different standards and have evolved no commonly accepted language.

The Advantage of a Treatment
That Avoids "Judging" Patients

Homeopathic physicians are lucky as we don't have to make these kinds of psychological judgments about our patients. Instead of dissecting our patients into various categories, homeopathic physicians think of them as physical, emotional and mental totalities. After all, the method of medicine-testing on healthy people which provides our *Materia Medica* lists the reactions of all these persons in their own everyday words. This "medicine picture" can then be applied directly to ill persons without first labeling them psychologically. Therefore, homeopathic physicians can focus on *treating* their psychological patients without first judging them! In other words, a homeopathic physician doesn't need first to decide if a patient is "depressed" or "excited" or "schizophrenic" or "psychopathic." or any other of the hundred and one labels placed by psychiatrists on their patients; labels differing by the "school" to which the psychiatrists belongs.

Rather, by considering the unanalyzed totality of a person's symptoms, a medicine specific to the *total* self can be found. And because the medicines' effects are expressed in everyday language and not in medical terminology, full allowance can be made for the *individual aptness* of a particular symptom expressed in everyday language. Thus, a whole complex illness may be unlocked by what is called in homeopathic practice a "rare, strange and peculiar" symptom.

A Method of Treating Paranoia

For instance, recently Miss Lois L., a 20-year old student, complained of "a splinter in her throat" when she swallowed. Although this might seem like nonsense, as we don't dine on wood, in homeopathy we have a number of medicines with this as a symptom. Thanks to this clue, I realized Lois needed a 12x dilution of silver nitrate, *Argentum nitricum*, for her combination of physical and emotional symptoms, her headache, frequent belching, apprehension on going into public places, restlessness, chilliness and female troubles. Within a few days she was herself.

Although it is not necessary (and is, in fact, often undesirable) for a homeopathic physician to differentiate between psychological patients—because the true psychotic patients are so dramatic, and in particular because ordinary medicine has so little to offer them—it might be interesting to consider a few examples of psychotic patients in my own practice. Obviously, I'm selecting a few who responded to homeopathic treatment and am not describing those who did not. However, any successes in this field are remarkable!

Fairly recently, Jane W., a young woman in her thirties, came to me for various intestinal problems. As we talked I soon became aware of her rigid personality. Almost casually she mentioned that her troubles followed persecution by a group of people who "had it in for her." They even had a machine which read her mind, providing them with information to use against her. After a few weeks of treatment particularly with barium carbonate, *Baryta carbonicum*, and the element Phosphorous in high dilutions, these delusions ceased to trouble her and she remained essentially free of them for the next two years. At about that time she moved away so that I have been out of touch.

Sophia F. came to me because certain people were trying to poison her with a foul gas which interfered with her breathing and made her exhausted. She has now been my patient for two years, and has received many medicines. She has no physical complaints of any significance and hasn't mentioned the poisoned gas for some time. However, she still insists that "people" are still doing things to her; such as injecting chemicals in her veins, so I can't say her delusions are cured. However, they have been modified, and her physical symptoms are certainly no longer present.

Of course, as I already pointed out, an accurate definition of the psychoneuroses is almost impossible. It is often more a social than a scientific definition, differing from social class to social class and even from country to country.

In the United States, older persons who have become confused or "crotchety" are often forcibly institutionalized because they have no one able, or willing, to care for them. Wealth make an enormous difference is such cases. Mrs. R., one of my patients in her eighties, is confused to the point where she can't handle her own finances and forgets what she said one minute before. However, she has a large private income as well as a wealthy family, so she is well taken care of. Another patient, Mrs. Z., of about the same age, is also confused and forgetful but she has no family and her husband is dead. Recently her confusion became worse than usual and was interspersed with episodes of suspicion about her landlady. Since no one could care for her during this acute episode she was placed in a mental hospital for a few months.

A Medicine Which Relieves Fear

How fortunate are homeopathic physicians that we are able to think in terms of "medicine pictures" rather than psychiatric labels. In other words, Billy G., a chilly, self-conscious boy who was fearful of everything and consistently performed far below the level of his abilities would be seen as needing a dose of sand, or Silica quartz, rather than classifying him as "inadequate," "hysterical," "neurotic," "father-dominated," or some other label which provides no practical method of therapy. Indeed, Silica 12x, over a 4-month period, removed all these symptoms. This manner of viewing disturbed persons also provides a handy method for differentiating between the many varied types of psychological problems people have—an ability to see the forest instead of the trees. Thus, homeopathic physicians see psychologically disturbed persons as needing high dilutions of Silica, or Sulfur, or Sepia or any one of thousands of other substances. This is a great comfort to the patient as well as the physician as it implies that the patient is lacking a certain energy pattern enclosed within the structure of a natural part of the universe—such as the anemome, *Pulsatilla,* or the oyster shell, *Calcarea ostrearum.* Viewed in this way, psychological illness can lose much of its strangeness and fear.

Much of psychological illness rises spontaneously with no readily apparent cause. Another group of psychological illnesses can be traced, at least in greater part, to some external cause. We might first consider this latter group as it is both familiar and readily understood.

How to Treat Grief and Despair with Medication

We have all of us, unfortunately, known grief; its first paroxysms of initial disbelief followed by weeping, a painful knot in the abdomen and a weakness as if all our strength has flown out of our limbs. This first stage of grief often responds to *Ignatia amara,* (St Ignatius Bean) in the 12x dilution, particularly when the grief is accompanied by involuntary sighing, oversensitivity to pain and a complete aversion to tobacco smoke.

Another outstanding medicine for grief is Phosphoric acid in high dilution. This grief is often from an unhappy love affair, homesickness or chagrin. Persons needing this medicine are prostrated from grief, uninterested in and cut off from the normal affairs of life and all those things once of interest. This is of particular value for elderly persons who have been prostrated from the loss of a life-long companion such as a husband or wife. I remember Roscoe H., an 80-year old widower whose dearly loved wife of 60 years had just died. Mr. H. became deeply depressed and withdrawn, mostly remaining in bed with his face to the wall. His children and grandchildren and life-time associates could not reach him. Phosphoric acid 12x quickly reduced his grief to more normal levels and restored him to his relatives and friends and his previous activities.

Despair and hopelessness commonly accompany grief, or they may come out of the blue for no apparent reason. In addition to Ignatia which we have already considered, there are some outstanding homeopathic medications for grief and hopelessness—in particular, *Aurum*, or gold. Interestingly enough, the organ in our bodies with the highest concentration of gold is the heart, and when our hearts are weak psychologically we know despair and hopelessness. Twenty-seven year old Richard T. suffered a hopelessness that verged on suicide. Life seemed a constant burden, and there was constant anxiety about the future. He was lethargic both physically and mentally, had a weak memory, and was easily fatigued; he was also chilly and suffered frequent palpitations. *Aurum* 12x relieved him in one week. In fact, the three other major remedies for hopelessness and despair are also chilly—*Psorinum, Arsenicum album* and *Calcarea ostrearum*. Of these three, psorinum is the most chilly. I will never forget Mrs. C., one of my Psorinum patients, who came to me on a sweltering August day wearing thermal underwear, a ski suit and a fur coat. And she was still chilly! After a month's treatment of Psorinum 12x she could wear more normal clothes.

With this Psorinum chilliness goes a hypersensitivity to drafts. Persons needing Psorinum both fear they will die and, at the same time, contemplate suicide. They are full of fears in general: of business failure, of religious salvation, of the future, and that they will never recover from their illness. These persons often have a bad odor—even just after a bath. It is a great medicine for hay fever and asthma, particularly when the asthma attacks appear less severe when lying flat in bed. Also, whenever a medicine which has been well selected doesn't help a person, or helps only temporarily, think of Psorinum. Psorinum is best purchased from a homeopathic pharmacy as you could not prepare it at home. The 12x dilution would be best.

Patients requiring *Arsenicum album*, along with despair and hopelessness have, like those needing Aurum and Psorinum, a great fear of death—so much so that it seems pointless to see a doctor or take any medicine because they are sure they will die. The hopelessness and fear is worse after midnight, particularly about 2 a.m. and is accompanied by great physical restlessness and anguish so that the Arsenicum patient will pace the room, back and forth, from wall to wall, showing at the same time an anguished fear-ridden expression. One of my patients, 45-year old Mrs. V., would leap out of bed each night at midnight and pace the floor until 2 a.m.,repeating "What's the use? I'm going to die! Why doesn't it come and finish me?" If her husband tried to comfort her she would irritably push him aside or throw things at him. After Arsenicum 12x she quieted down and became normal. Although chilly, these patients crave cold water which they sip like a cat, a little at a time but frequently. If patients requiring Arsenicum have pain it is a burning pain, like fire, as if hot coals had been touched to the part affected.

The *Calcarea ostrearum* depression is more like its namesake, the oyster—a big, fat, stationary depression, in which the person is immobilized by fear and melancholy. Joan S., an 18-year old, suffered this. She didn't move around like the Arsenicum people, but just sat, drowning in her own melancholy. In addition to feeling chilly internally, Joan felt cold and clammy to another's touch. Full of fears—of disease, disaster, insanity, being observed by others, etc.—she was immobilized by fear; she was cautious, confused, sad, apathetic, even misplacing words as she spoke. In two weeks, *Calcarea ostrearum* 6x relieved her symptoms. Mrs. Andre S., a 50-year old decorator, was greatly helped by a 12x dilution of another great remedy for hopelessness and despair, the tiger lily, *Lilium tigrinum*. Who would think such a dramatically colorful and boldly cheerful flower would be full of despair and insanity? Like the tiger and, indeed, all the members of the cat family, people in need of *Lilium tigrinum* swing widely from mood to mood. At times profoundly depressed, timid, fearful and constantly weeping, they may as suddenly curse, use obscene language and strike out at those around them. Full of paradoxes, they are listless, but cannot sit still, restless, but averse to walking, desire to do something—indeed hurry to do it—yet have no ambition. Sometimes these are persons who keep busy to repress their sexual desires.

With its left-sidedness and action on the female organs, this medicine often complements the action of the great woman's remedy, Sepia. Indeed, I think of it as my "crazy Sepia" medicine for hysterical women, acting like Scarlet O'Hara in *Gone with the Wind*.

Remedies for Anger

Anger is another common, troubling psychological problem. Homeopathy has a number of extremely effective medicines for this, both for angry, irritable persons and for persons made sick from the effects of anger. Outstanding among them are the Wild Hop, *Bryonia alba*, the herb *Chamomilla*, the Wolf's Foot, *Lycopodium*, the herb *Nux vomica*, and Stavesacre, *Staphisagria*. Persons needing Bryonia and Nux vomica have many characteristics in common. They are often slender brunettes with dark complexions. Many tense, excitable persons from the Mediterranean area, or of Mediterranean origins, need these remedies—the Spanish, Southern French and the Italians. My first Bryonia patient was John B., son of my Italian-American landlord. He was tense, irritable and constantly angry, so that he made life miserable for his family. He also had another outstanding Bryonia symptom in that he lost interest whenever he was given what he asked for and immediately wanted something else. One dose of Bryonia 12x dilution returned him to normal in one week.

Bryonia complaints follow cold drinks or cold food in hot weather, whereas Nux vomica complaints are worse after spicy foods or coffee, tobacco or alcohol. They both are better from rest and worse on motion, Bryonia in particular. Bryonia patients are thirsty for large quantities at long intervals of time; and Bryonia has the peculiar symptom that painful parts are better if lain upon. As Nux vomica features neither of these two symptoms, they serve as a means of differentiating between the two medicines. Further, patients requiring Nux vomica are hypersensitive to their environment, particularly to noises, odors, light or music, and they are full of gastric complaints, in particular gas or nausea after meals. As usual, Nux vomica in the 12x dilution often helps these symptoms.

As Bryonia shares certain symptoms in common with Nux vomica, so does it with Staphisagria. Both Bryonia and Staphisagria are worse from the results of anger (Bryonia people are also angry people; Staphisagria, less so). Staphisagria is good for persons such as a 40-year old accountant in my practice, Mr. W., who was indignant over past grievances. He was as sensitive to emotional hurt as Nux vomica is to physical stimuli—full of ailments from excessive pride, envy or chagrin. Like Bryonia, he lost interest in what he previously asked for, always wanting something new. I have had many spoiled children in my practice who benefitted from this medicine. Whereas patients requiring Nux vomica will blow up at the slightest irritation, making everyone around them miserable, the Staphisagria patient is too dignified to fight and instead swallows his anger and goes home sick, trembling and exhausted with suppressed anger. A 6x dilution of Staphisagria greatly helped Mr. W. in a few days. Staphisagria is also useful for mechanical injuries from sharp instruments.

The remaining two medicines for anger, *Chamomilla* and *Lycopodium*, are for persons whose anger is more a superficial peevishness and irritability than a deep emotion. The Lycopodium patient often has an overdeveloped mind, so that he is constantly criticizing others, even going out of his way to start arguments. As is often the case with bullies, this patient can't stand opposition or contradiction of any kind. Yet, in spite of his being miserable to people around him, the patient requiring Lycopodium can't stand to be alone and is forced constantly to seek company. The Chamomilla patient is also peevish and fretful. This is the great medicine for babies, particularly teething babies, who cry constantly if put down and are quiet only when carried. I must have given it in the 6x dilution to hundreds of teething babies through the years for this single symptom, usually with relief.

5

Homeopathic Relief for Female Troubles

Adult women often have problems unique to their menses and pregnancy. The illnesses of boys and girls differ little from one another before puberty save that girls in general seem to be healthier, huskier, more mature and better at school work than their masculine counterparts. Boys suffer more injuries from accidents, as any parent knows.

With the onset of her menstrual period, a girl starts the physical and emotional up and down life she will know at least until the menopause and possibly for years after it. It's no wonder the boys start to catch up with the girls in adolescence.

The Problems That Constitute Woman's Most Common Trouble

From the onset of her menses, a woman becomes a creature of the moon, swayed by the ebbing and flowing of the hormonal tide in her blood. Some women can go a lifetime without any menstrual problems, but, at least in this country, that is not true for the average woman. In fact, for many women menstrual problems are the most frequent form of disability.

As no woman wants to wear a hat or dress like that worn by another woman, so do women react in an individual way to their menstrual problems. Some are worse before, some during and some after the menses. Other are better during their menses. Some have pains in the back, others in the front, some around the left ovary, some around the right ovary, etc. Thus there are almost as many patterns of menstrual irregularities as there are women experiencing them. Because of the many hundreds of available homeopathic medicines, each with its varied, individual application, these many different reactions to the menses can usually be treated by one homeopathic medicine or another. However, such a recounting of medications suitable for women's menstrual problems becomes almost a textbook in itself, completely unsuited to a home treatment book such as this. Therefore, I have selected a few of the outstanding 'women's remedies' for our joint consideration, omitting literally hundreds of important medications, in the process.

The Most Effective Homeopathic Medicine for All Female Trouble

The outstanding homeopathic medicine for menstrual difficulties is certainly the ink and the ground up enclosing sac of the common ocean-living squid, known scientifically as *Sepia officinalis*. This benign looking brownish ink is able, at least potentially, to offer relief for virtually all of the common illnesses of women.

It relieves a whole spectrum of menstrual difficulties—menses too long, too short, too profuse, too scanty, too frequent, too infrequent, clotted or too thin. It may relieve any complaint from any part of the body which is worse before the menses. It relieves pressing, bearing-down pains of the female organs which feel as if everything would fall out of the pelvis. Often a woman needing Sepia will sit with her legs crossed or held tightly together because she is convinced her internal organs will fall out if she doesn't do so.

In addition to menstrual difficulties, Sepia is good for all phases of a woman's hormonal life. It helps establish the menses properly in young girls who have irregular, scanty periods. Later on, in pregnancy, Sepia is of value for sterility, for frequent miscarriage during the first three months of pregnancy, and for morning sickness of pregnancy when the smell of food, or even the thought of food, is nauseating. It is helpful for car sickness from pregnancy or any other cause.

Sepia's value in frequent miscarriage can be dramatic. Mrs. Sandra R., a pregnant actress in her early thirties came to me with a sad history of six previous miscarriages all in the first three months of pregnancy. Other than this, she presented the typical Sepia picture of chilliness, menstrual irregularities, depression, etc. After one dose of Sepia 12x Sandra stopped staining (she was then two months pregnant and had been staining for the entire two months). Much to her surprise and delight, for the first time her pregnancy continued beyond the third month and, although she did stain again periodically during the pregnancy she went to full term and had a little girl, normal in every way. Within a year or so she became pregnant again, and again went to term, producing a healthy boy.

Later, in middle-life, a need for Sepia presents (as did 45-year old Polly R.,) the picture of the typical harrassed housewife: sallow, chilly, depressed and complaining, constantly tired—an hysterical tyrant before her menses and between her menses irritable and unhappy with her home and family. As this kind of woman alienates everyone in touch with her, in addition to rapidly restoring Polly's physical and emotional health, administration of Sepia 6x renewed a happy life for the whole family.

Later on, when a woman enters the menopause, Sepia can again help, this time with hot flashes, the pain on intercourse, and the general insanity which so often accompanies the menopause.

Sepia is the woman's remedy par excellence. I probably give it to three quarters of my women patients at one time or another. One of my old teachers once told me half in jest that he could practice homeopathy with three remedies—Sepia for the ladies, Sulfur for the men and Arnica for injuries. Sometimes when I view my own practice I think he was right. Since you probably cannot get a squid from your local grocery store, probably you had best obtain your Sepia (in the 6x or 12x) from a homeopathic pharmacy. One dose of the 6x is best to start treatment, followed, if necessary, by two other doses at 24-hour intervals. If the 6x doesn't help after a few days, you can repeat with the 12x.

A Particularly Helpful Medication for Problems of Young Girls

Regardless of how much Sepia I use I still need many other medicines for female troubles. Another medicine for girls when their menses first appear is the Anemone, *Pulsatilla nigercans*. If Sepia is the woman's remedy, Pulsatilla is the girl's remedy. Nancy M., a 13-

year old, was typical of patients in needs of Pulsatilla. Nancy was mild, gentle, timid and of a yielding disposition, slow in physical and mental activity, and easily moved to laughter or to tears. She cried so easily it often interfered with her recounting her symptoms to me. Like many young girls, Nancy was fickle, constantly changing her mind. Even her symptoms changed constantly—no two chills, no two attacks were ever the same. Also, her menses were irregular, sometimes present, other times not. Nancy was well one minute and sick the next. Her pains came and went rapidly shifting from one place to another. I prescribed Pulsatilla 12x, one dose in a.m. and p.m. for two days. Relief soon followed. Although I obtain my Pulsatilla from a homeopathic pharmacy, it could be made from an alcoholic tincture of the fresh flower, following the directions given in Chapter 1.

Pulsatilla is specific for problems at the onset of the menses, when the first menstruation is delayed, or if established it is intermittent, coming and going irregularly, or suppressed after wet feet. Pulsatilla is also helpful in threatened miscarriages, when the menstrual flow ceases and then returns with increased force, with spasmodic pains which suffocate the patient, who is always better with lots of fresh air. In addition to a marked improvement in the fresh air, Pulsatilla patients are made worse in a warm room or by fatty foods, and, although complaining of a dry mouth in the morning they are thirstless at all times.

Another Highly Effective Remedy for Female Problems

The third of the great woman's remedies is the common Birthwort, or the Long Aristolochy as it is sometimes called. Its botanical name is *Aristolochia clematatis,* from the Greek *aristos,* meaning "best," and *lochia,* meaning "childbirth." It is an ancient medicine and, as its name implies, its value in childbirth has long been appreciated. It seems to blend many of the characteristics of Sepia and Pulsatilla. It is useful in the female genital tract when the menses are lost, delayed, or too long or too short. (It is also helpful in problems of the male genital tract such as inflammation of the prostate or the epididymis.) Illnesses connected with the genital tract such as menopausal arthritis, sterility, labor and gonorrhea also often respond. It is one of the first medicines to think of for vaginal discharges (leucorrhea) of all kinds, often white or of a brown, slimy character, accompanied by severe itching and sexual desire.

It has the pre-menstrual aggravation of Sepia combined with the alternation between sad and happy moods or between introversion and extroversion of Pulsatilla. In addition to its genital action it is an outstanding medicine for urinary tract inflammations, varicose veins, gastric upsets and skin conditions.

I have given the symptom picture of Sepia, Pulsatilla and Aristolochia in some detail to show their broad range of action. Since they are all three useful for similar conditions you might ask how can I tell if I need one or the other? Here is where the art of homeopathy comes in, showing its particular strength. In addition to thinking of your menstrual symptoms, you must not forget your general, nonmenstrual picture.

Thus, if you are predominantly a chilly person with cold hands and feet, who likes warmth and avoids cold, who likes the doors and windows closed, and has a tendency to be gassy and constipated, then Sepia may be the medicine for you.

On the other hand, if you tend to be warm, better in the fresh air and wishing the doors and windows open, even in the winter, and of a gentle, sometimes too good-natured disposition, easily moved to tears from the troubles of others—even sad movies or TV programs—then your medicine is Pulsatilla.

Thus we have differentiated between two medicines which have a similar action on the menses. Since Aristolochia combines the qualities and actions of both Sepia and Pulsatilla, I use it as a backstop remedy when the other two medications have not done the trick.

If one or another of these three medicines doesn't help, you might wish to consider some others. Again, out of the medley of hundreds of medicines available for your particular menstrual difficulty, we must focus on only a few of the most common.

Relieving Painful Menstruation

For painful menses, in general, the common garden herb Chamomilla may help, particularly if you feel peevish, impatient and don't want to be spoken to, or have anyone near you.

If your pain is greatest on the right side, is like a dragging and pressing downwards which starts in your back and spreads to your front, the common garden herb Nightshade, or Belladonna, may give you relief. If the pain is also of a dragging down nature but worse on the *left* side, particularly if you are weepy, irritable or worse in other ways a few days before your period, then the ink of the squid, Sepia, may help. Victoria B., suffered pains so extreme that they seemed unendurable. Since she was also overweight, a 6x dilution of the common herb Monkshood (*Aconitum napellus*) helped. Natalie W. suffered pains (particularly pains of a squeezing and constricting nature) so acute that she cried out, so I gave her one dose of a 12x dilution of the desert flower, *Cactus grandiflora*, which gave her relief.

How to Treat Heavy Periods

Possibly your menses are too heavy. If your previous period was normal, and this one seems normal but just much heavier, then you may need a little iron in homeopathic form, called *Ferrum metallicum*. This is particularly indicated if your face seems unusually pale—even your lips and gums—but you become bright red on the least pain, emotion or exertion. On the other hand, if the whole character of your menses seems changed, with profuse bleeding of bright red blood, often full of clots, particularly if they are accompanied by nausea and vomiting, try the South American herb Ipecac. This is of value even for bright red bleeding between your periods. In the section on intestinal problems I already mentioned the ready availability of Ipecac tincture at any drugstore and explained how you add one drop of Ipecac tincture to 10 drops of ethyl alcohol and hit its containing bottle 15 times against your palm. Repeat this process six times and you have prepared the 6x dilution.

If your flow is profuse and bright red but is better if you walk or stand, then the herb Savine, or Sabina, may give you relief, particularly if you have drawing pains from the small of your back extending downwards to your pelvis. If your flow is dark, with discomfort in your ovaries, ordinary Witch Hazel, *Hamamelis virginica*, may help. This you can probably get in the tincture form from your local drugstore, which you can then make into a medicine if you wish. Be sure not to get the Witch Hazel combined with rubbing alcohol as rubbing alcohol is poisonous. If your periods are dark and full of black lumps, particularly if you are full of gas and have shaking chills, you may need quinine, or Cinchona, also available from your local drugstore. As it is soluble in water, you can easily make it up into a medicine should you wish to do so.

How to Treat Delayed and Scanty Menses

On the other hand, if your menses are delayed and scanty, accompanied by flushing, skin eruptions, and a faint sinking feeling before lunch, consider the element Sulfur. Or if they are scanty and delayed and you are worse from heat in general, particularly from the sun, and if you crave salty food and are constipated, then ordinary table salt, *Natrum muriaticum*, may help. As this is as near as your pantry and is readily soluble in water, you can easily make some up for your own use. If in addition to being scanty and delayed, your periods are black and tarry and flow only when you lie down, ceasing when you walk around, particularly if accompanied by sour belching and heart burn, then magnesia carbonate, *Magnesia carbonica*—which you know as Milk of Magnesia—may help. Again, as this is readily available to you, you can "roll" your own.

And, finally, if your period is delayed because you were chilled (this is common in young girls whose periods are not fully established) the common Monkshood, *Aconitum napellus*, may help.

Medicines for Pregnancy

Pregnancy, an important point in any woman's life, is also an ideal time for homeopathic treatment as the medicines can influence both the mother and her baby simultaneously. In fact, a pregnant woman's symptoms are usually a combination of her own symptoms of pregnancy and of the symptoms of the baby she is carrying. I have seen this over and over as I compare the symptoms of each child with those of the mother during pregnancy, varying from pregnancy to pregnancy.

In addition, during pregnancy a woman will often respond better to homeopathic treatment than at any other time as she usually avoids anything—like medicines, alcohol, tobacco, etc.—which might interfere with her babies' health. Many of these substances also interfere with homeopathic treatment.

I have always been struck by women's—even nonpregnant women's—greater sensitivity to external things such as the odor of paint, chemical sprays, foods, insect bites, and countless other environmental factors. I am convinced that this greater sensitivity of women provides a protection for the children they carry within themselves. Indeed, modern research has shown that babies in uteri are sensitive to everything which affects the mother. This confirms the correctness of many "old wives tales" which advise pregnant women to avoid fresh paint odors, alcohol, coffee, etc. Therefore, husbands, fathers and male physicians should honor and respect these feminine sensitivities as preserving the health of the race, rather than becoming impatient with what seems to masculine ears "female nonsense."

For all this complex of reasons, the homeopathic treatment of pregnant women is uniquely desirable and effective, both for the mother and her offspring.

Relief of Morning Sickness

Among the specific complaints of pregnancy, morning sickness is one of the most frequent. The first medicine I think of for this condition is the squid, Sepia. If food is vomited as soon as it hits the stomach and you have a lot of gas and feel chilly and irritable, the herb Nux vomica may help. Another indicator for Nux vomica is a brown coated tongue. If it is moist and white and the morning sickness is worse after fats and better in fresh air, use Pulsatilla, the anemone. If Nux vomica doesn't help, you might try calcium flouride, *Calcarea fluorica*. It is a great help for all types of digestive troubles in pregnancy and also helps delivery if it is given in the last few months of pregnancy.

If the nausea continues day and night without vomiting try tobacco, *Tabacum*, whose preparation was described in the section on intestinal troubles.

Remedies for Heartburn

Next to morning sickness, heartburn is a frequent complaint of pregnancy. (By heartburn is meant a burning in the center of the chest underneath the breast bone, often extending to the left to include the region of the heart.) For simple heartburn Pulsatilla, or red pepper, *Capsicum*, often brings relief. If it is combined with a sour taste in the mouth, try *Calcarea ostrearum* ground oyster shell.

The Treatment of Food Cravings in Pregnancy

As most fathers know, pregnant ladies develop the strangest food craving, often in the small hours of the morning. These are so varied they would require a separate chapter by themselves, particularly because the full and complex homeopathic *Materia Medica* provides literally hundreds of medicines to treat these dietary peculiarities. However, we can consider a few of the most common ones.

The classic pregnancy desire is for pickles or other sour things. I think this is because so many women (at least in this country) need Sepia, and Sepia has a great desire for sour things. A desire for sweets is also common. Here you might consider the element Sulfur or, if you are very gassy, the Wolf's Foot, *Lycopodium clavatum*. If you wish salty things, you may need charcoal, *Carbo vegetabilis* (particularly if you are full of gas) or common table salt, *Natrum muriaticum*, (particularly if you can't stand the sun, and want to be by yourself).

Urinary frequency is another common complaint of pregnancy. For simple urinary urging think of homeopathic dilutions of deadly Nightshade, Belladonna, or Nux vomica or Pulsatilla which are already mentioned. If it is accompanied by burning or scalding, consider Spanish Fly, *Cantharis*, or if urine leaks out on the slightest exertion or after coughing or sneezing, consider *Causticum*.

Backache is another common problem in pregnancy. If you have weakness and a dragging feeling in the loins think of potassium carbonate, *Kali carbonicum*, or if the back feels bruised and you walk with difficulty, try *Bellis perennis*, the common daisy. As already described you can prepare your own medicine by crushing a fresh daisy in ethyl alcohol and placing one drop of the tincture with 9 drops of ethyl alcohol in a separate bottle. Strike the bottle against your palm 15 times and add one drop of this mixture to 9 drops of ethyl alcohol. Continue the process six times and you have a 6x dilution.

And finally, if your breasts are painful, try Hemlock, *Conium maculatum*, or the wild hop, *Bryonia alba*, and if you have cramps in your calves which prevent sleep, try a 12x dilution of coffee, *Coffea cruda*, or Nux vomica.

How to Treat Menopausal Troubles

At the other end of the time scale, when a woman moves into her change of life (menopause) every part of her body is affected—physical, emotional and mental, although some women, of course, go through the menopause without a symptom. My two most successful medicines for menopause are the South American Surukuku snake venom, *Lachesis*, and the ink from the squid, *Sepia*. They both are used for hot flashes and irritability but if you are worse in the morning, can't stand heat and are hypersensitive to the least pressure so that tight clothing is intolerable, then Lachesis is indicated, but if, by contrast, you are worse in the evening, can't stand the cold and are weepy and despondent, then Sepia is for you. If Sepia doesn't help, then you may need Sulfuric acid to complete the action of Sepia. If you are irritable, depressed and sleepless and also have a feeling of a ball in your throat then the old folk remedy for nervous ladies, Valerian, may help. (You can get this in any herb shop, and many gardens, for your home preparation). Or, if you have a feeling of a ball in your throat and are nervous, depressed, constipated and have numbness in various places and a sinking sensation in the pit of your stomach, then St. Ignatius' bean, *Ignatia*, may give you relief.

Lastly, I must not forget to mention Plumbago, or *Graphites*, which is as specific for menopause as Pulsatilla is for girls at puberty. If you need Graphites you will be constipated, timid and sad, and like Sepia, often not interested in sex, and the sound of music may make you weep. Since Graphites is the "lead" used in pencils, you should have no trouble acquiring some if you wish to make your own medication.

6

Easing Your Allergies with Homeopathic Treatment

Why So Many of Us Are Allergic

As we all know, allergies are unusual reactions to things which most people either don't react to at all, or react to in a predictable, common manner. According to many authorities, allergies are becoming more frequent all the time, possibly because our environment is becoming more complex each year, exposing us to new and different foods and chemicals we're not used to. For instance, people from parts of the world where cow's milk is not used—like Equatorial Africa and most of Asia except India—are much more frequently allergic to cow's milk than are those of us from Europe and North America, where it is often the first food we move to from mother's milk. Some authorities say that many of the new chemicals, when added to our foods, produce allergies by destroying our protective mechanisms, thus decreasing our abilities to deal with new substances in our environment. Other authorities say that our unhealthy eating and living habits have produced our increased sensitivities, and that they disappear when we eat properly.

Whatever the reason, allergies are a serious health problem in the United States today, accounting for hundreds of millions of hours of sickness each year, with the loss of industrial productivity and the personal expense that all this implies.

As is generally known, allergies are usually treated by first finding the causative agent and then either avoiding it or else undergoing a series of injections of high dilutions of this causative agent in an attempt to "desensitize" us to it. This is certainly a useful technique, and can often help. By this method of serial exposure to dilute agents immunity can even be built in to poisons. Ancient kings, in fear of poison, often built up immunity to many poisons by starting each day off with a drink of diluted poisons. In like manner, young boys in the Hopi Indian snake cult are started off with frequent bites from baby rattlesnakes, until they can tolerate the poison of a full-grown rattler.

Homeopathic medicines also have a great deal to offer in the treatment of allergies. They operate in several ways. Most commonly the allergic symptoms are treated with substances which would produce them in the healthy. This represents an "individualization" of the patient to his or her particular symptoms, since our reactions to an allergic substance may differ from each other. For instance, Joan S., one of my patients, a young girl of eight, turns red and looks like a tomato if she eats tomatoes. Joan usually develops a cough, which will hang on for weeks, and loses her sense of balance so that she frequently falls. Henry, her father, on the other hand, gets a bloody crust in his nose and congestion of his frontal sinuses if he eats tomatoes. Each one needed a different homeopathic medicine for their tomato allergy—Sulfur 6x for Joan and Sepia 12x for Henry—and, after one year of treatment their tomato allergies disappeared.

Homeopathic Desensitization

Sometimes it is found more effective to treat the allergy directly with a homeopathic preparation of the agent which caused it. For instance, some persons who are allergic to poison ivy can be helped to lose their sensitivity if, in the spring, before the poison ivy comes up, they take one dose of an extremely high homeopathic dilution of the poison ivy plant (*Rhus toxicodendron*). I have had great success with this. The majority of patients who took Rhus tox in homeopathic dilution have lost their poison ivy sensitivity. Bill F., in particular, comes to mind. He was on a highway maintenance gang and every spring and summer for years had contracted ivy poisoning. One dose of Rhus tox 12x each February keeps Bill clear for the year. If you are unfortunate enough to be allergic to poison ivy, I strongly recommend that you immunize yourself with Rhus tox 12x before the next season comes along. This one tip should more than repay the time and money you have spent on this book. Allergies to poison oak (*Rhus diversiloba*), poison sumach (*Rhus glabra*) and other botanical poisons can often be prevented in a similar manner.

Thus, there are two methods in general of treating allergies homeopathically—by using the individual symptoms of the sufferer as a guide to the medicine (individualizing the patient) or by giving the allergic material in homeopathic dilution (desensitizing the patient). This latter method works best where there is a clear-cut history of allergy to a single substance. When allergies are multiple, as is frequently true, then the classic method of homeopathic "individualization" can often remove the basic sensitivity to the various allergic substances. Helen W., a 25-year old secretary, had ragweed hay fever each fall, sinusitis from milk and eczema from wheat. As she was chilly and worse before her periods I gave her Sepia 12x which helped the chilliness and periods and also *removed* her allergies.

Incidentally, a homeopathic preparation of any substance can be prepared for you by any homeopathic pharmacy. Through the years I have acquired some peculiar desensitizing medicines—green peas, egg white, cat dander, etc. As I mentioned in Chapter 3, I even had a tick preparation made up for me for a young girl who developed a bald spot on her scalp at a point where a tick bit her!

How You Can Mix Your Own Medicines

If you can't wait for a special desensitizing medicine to be made up for you by a homeopathic pharmacy, you can make your own. If your sensitive agent is water- or alcohol-soluble you can prepare a medicine from it by mixing it thoroughly in an 87% ethyl alcohol and water solution. (If it is *not* soluble in an alcohol-water mixture you should have it prepared by a homeopathic pharmacist.) Add one drop of this first mixture to a separate bottle containing 9 drops of the 87% ethyl alcohol-water mixture. Strike this second bottle sharply 15 times against a leather shoe, your thigh, or any other firm but soft object which won't shatter the glass. This is called 'succussion' by pharmacists. (Obviously, get bottles with thick sides for this work!) Place one drop from bottle No. 2 into a similar bottle (No.3) containing nine drops of the alcohol and water mixture and repeat the process. Continue in this manner from bottle to bottle until you have used either six or twelve bottles other than the one with the initial tincture in it. In this manner you have prepared a sixth or twelfth serial dilution. You can keep all the dilutions you prepared, but in light-resistant brown bottles with neutral plastic, cork, or glass tops which will not enter into chemical action with the contents.

When you use these medicines on yourself for allergy treatment, start with the highest dilution (6x or 12x) to avoid any adverse reaction. The usual dose is one drop of the medicine in a glass of water. Take one sip from the glass and note its effect. If you are better, stop there. If there has been no effect, take another sip in three hours, and repeat again in three hours if necessary. If you still have noticed no change in your symptoms you can try taking one sip each morning for a week, as some cases are more stubborn than others. If no change has occurred after a week, then you had best stop the whole procedure.

If you noticed a change, discontinue the medicine. If your symptoms return repeat the treatment procedure already outlined, immediately stopping the medicine when you note a change.

Some fortunate persons will find that their symptoms will disappear permanently under the preceding treatment. They are, hopefully, cured of their allergy. Others will find that their symptoms have improved, but return when they discontinue the medication. This represents a palliation, not a cure, and indicates that a deeper homeopathic treatment or possibly another type of treatment is necessary for a cure, if, indeed, a cure is possible. In the meantime, relief of the symptoms can be continued, no mean blessing in itself, and of particular value for seasonal allergies like hay fever.

Incidentally, before making your own desensitizing medication you might check with one of the homeopathic pharmacists as to what they have in stock. Many of them carry a large selection of common allergic substances, such as ragweed, poison ivy, DDT, and so on.

So much for our necessarily rather superficial consideration of the preparation and use of specific homeopathic allergic desensitizing medicines. Now, how do you go about treating your allergic symptoms by relating them individually to the symptoms produced on healthy persons by various substances—substances completely unrelated to the apparent cause of your allergy? For instance, spring hay fever caused by tree or rose pollens is often helped by homeopathic dilution of *Allium cepa*, the common onion.

First, we will consider the common allergies like asthma, hay fever and hives, relating to the part affected by the allergy. Then we will consider the allergies determined by environment, such as allergies to articles of clothing or food. In this latter group you may find new, specific, homeopathic concepts of particular interest to you.

Hay Fever Medicines

Respiratory allergies probably make up the most common group of allergies. Most of us know that hay fever and asthma are usually allergic in cause. Less of us know that repeated colds and sinus trouble are frequently allergic. The old saying "If you sneeze more than five times, or if your cold lasts more than a week, it is an allergy," is often true.

First of all, let's consider that seasonal bug-a-boo so familiar to many of us, hay fever. As I already mentioned, the common onion, *Allium cepa*, is frequently of value in hay fever, worse in the spring or fall. We are all familiar with how we feel when we peel an onion—the running, burning eyes and nose, and the profuse, watery and acrid nasal discharge. These symptoms are of course very like those many of us have when we have hay fever. They are also high in importance among the symptoms developed by healthy persons when they take *Allium cepa* as part of a contrived homeopathic testing under the supervision of homeopathic physician. Other symptoms are frequently produced as part of this homeopathic testing. These symptoms, also included in the "picture" of *Allium cepa* as used by homeopathic physicians, are a dull headache, worse in the evening, better in the open air and worse on returning to a warm room. There is also violent sneezing on first getting out of bed, or from handling peaches. Also, there are colicky abdominal pains often following wet feet, cucumbers, salads or overeating.

I have found the onion in high dilution to be my single most effective medication for spring and fall hay fever, and, as it is as close as your nearest grocery store, you can readily prepare your own medication by dilution and agitation of the alcoholic tincture to the 6x and 12x dilutions. Joseph W., a 25-year old teacher, each spring suffered acute sneezing, running eyes, and a dull headache, which was better in the fresh air. He prepared some *Allium cepa* 12x under my direction, and he is now free of his springtime hay fever.

Joan N., a 32-year old night club dancer, had an attack of hay fever brought on by exposure to cold, damp, rainy weather, and a sudden change from hot to cold weather. As *Dulcamara* (the Bittersweet) fitted these symptoms, I gave her a 12x dilution which gave her relief in a few hours.

If children (or grownups) suffer hay fever after wading in cold water in bare feet, think of *Dulcamara*. As *Dulcamara* grows in many gardens, should you care to do so you can readily prepare your own dilution, in the manner already described.

If brought on in the summer by overexposure to the sun or intense heat, think of *Natrum muriaticum*, common salt.

People who need *Natrum muriaticum* act as if they had lost their salt. They are weepy for no reason, irritable, scrawny, constipated, and crave salt. They can't stand the sun or the atmosphere at the seaside—even indoors at the seashore they are worse. I remember Anne S., a middle-aged housewife, whose husband was a beach nut. Every summer Anne dutifully dragged herself to the beach where she spent the summer sniffing and blowing like a porpoise. Come fall when she went home all her symptoms miraculously vanished, even though she returned in September which was the height of the inland ragweed season. After a dose of *Natrum muriaticum* 12x (salt) she was able to enjoy her summer at the beach for the first time in her memory. Isn't it interesting that Mrs. S. was worse at the beach surrounded by salt water, yet it was that very salt in homeopathic dilution which was able to restore her health. This illustrates how differently a substance acts in gross dosage, compared to its action after special preparation via homeopathic serial dilution and succession.

Incidentally, although out of place at this point, I can't resist telling of another effective use of *Natrum muriaticum*, but not in homeopathic potency. Ordinary salt seems to be specific for the treatment of acute poison ivy poisoning. I was first tipped off to this by an old gardener who said that if he got a little patch of poison ivy he immediately rubbed ordinary table salt on it. In most cases that took care of it for him. I passed this tip on to my patients and many of them said it worked.

Another tip I learned a few summers ago from Mr. John T., a patient who spent the summer at an ocean beach which was literally festooned in poison ivy—even the boardwalk along the beach had tendrils sticking up in the cracks between the boards, ready to poison any bare foot which passed by. John was convinced that he would get poison ivy but the local residents insisted that no one on the island ever got it as long as they bathed in the salt water each day. He didn't believe them, but decided to give it a whirl, not only swimming each day, but not bathing in fresh water on shore. As he said, "By the end of the visit I was smelly, and my hair looked like a haystack, but I had no poison ivy!" Since then, I send patients with acute ivy poisoning to the nearest salt water beach, usually with good results. Just bathing at home in a tub of cold water saturated with rock salt does seem to help, but the real salt water seems to be specific. Please excuse the digression; now back to hay fever.

If the sneezing comes in paroxysms, followed by watering from the eyes and nose (like *Allium cepa*), accompanied by a hot face and red, burning eyelids and dryness of the skin, throat and tonsillar area, think of the herb *Sabadilla*. If this grows in your garden, you can crush it in alcohol and add one drop of this herbal tincture to nine drops of alcohol in a separate bottle. Hit the bottle 15 times against your palm, as already described, then repeat the process until you have a 6x or 12x dilution, to use on yourself.

And finally, if the hay fever returns every year on the same day of the month, and there is a previous history of asthma or eczema think of administering a homeopathic dose of the skin parasite, *Psorinum*. Patients needing *Psorinum* are so chilly and sensitive to cold air that they will wear a fur coat or cap even in the hottest weather. *Psorinum* is most effective in *preventing* hay fever, if given a number of months before the attack is due. Like other homeopathic medicines made from disease organisms you had best purchase *Psorinum* from a homeopathic pharmacy, rather than try to make it yourself.

Asthma Medicines

Asthma is another allergic misery. It is usually more of a chronic disease than hay fever as it is less subject to seasonal changes, although some unfortunates with hay fever also have asthma as part of their troubles. As most of us know, asthma and hay fever—and indeed all allergies—tend to run in families. If both parents are allergic it's hard for their children to escape it. In my experience hay fever is largely an adult disease. Asthma, on the other hand, seems to affect both children and adults equally.

Children with eczema in their early years may develop asthma in their teens. Homeopathic physicians find that this often follows treatment of the eczema with cortisone, X-rays, or skin salves of one sort or another—as if denying the eczema illness a place on the skin drives it inward to settle on the lungs. Repeatedly, homeopathic physicians have to reestablish an old eczema (often forgotten by the sufferer) before a stubborn case of asthma will clear up.

Among allergic asthma medicines, the traditional American Indian herb, Indian turnip (*Arum triphyllum*) is one of the best. In addition to the asthma there is usually a profuse, acrid nasal discharge which irritates the lining of and the inside of the nose and the upper lip. There is an irresistible urge to pick at the nose and lips until they bleed. Often accompanying this is a hoarse uncertain voice, worse from talking and singing, sometimes ending in a complete voice loss. You can prepare your own medicine from one drop of the fresh herb in alcoholic tincture added to nine drops of alcohol. Hit the containing bottle 15 times against your hand and continue the dilution in the usual manner to the 6x and 12x.

If the asthma is worse after midnight and worse lying down, better by leaning forward in bed with the chest against the thighs or walking around the room, then *Arsenicum album* (the white oxide of arsenic, arsenic trioxide) is often useful. This asthma is usually made worse by cold drinks. These patients, either depressed or indifferent to everything, are often anxious, and irritable. They are afraid they will die, or that their disease is incurable. Their agitation is combined with an unbelievable physical restlessness. I remember Mrs. Nadine B., a swarthy, middle-aged singer who came to me with a long history of allergic asthma attacks. Each night at midnight, on the dot, her asthma attacks would start, always with the same pattern. Nadine would leap out of bed and start pacing the room, at the same time wheezing, crying, shivering (even in the hot, muggy August night when she first came to me) and calling to her husband to be with her, as she was about to die. This classic picture naturally led me to give her *Arsenicum album* 12x which put things straight in a few minutes, much to the relief of the patient and her husband.

The halogen family of chemical elements have an interesting relationship with allergies. We have already discussed chlorine, in the form of its sodium salt, sodium chloride (or *Natrum muriaticum*) in its relationship to hay fever.

Iodine and bromine, two other halogen gases, in high dilutions are of value in asthma. In contradistinction to *Natrum muriaticum* with its hay fever at the seaside, *Bromium* is of value for sailors who develop asthma as soon as they go ashore. It acts best on persons with light-blue eyes, flaxen hair, light eyebrows and a fair, delicate skin. *Iodum*, by constrast, is particularly indicated for persons with dark hair and eyes. It is the typical case of overactive thyroid (this can be produced by excess iodine intake) with ravenous hunger while losing weight constantly, great emaciation, palpitations, sensitivity to heat, constipation, and profound weakness. The asthma attacks of Iodum patients are much worse in warm rooms, and better in cool air. Interestingly, both Iodum and Bromium have the sensation "as if the heart is clasped and unclasped rapidly by an iron hand." As both Iodine and Bromine are toxic gases, you will not be able to prepare them at home but must get them from a homeopathic pharmacy.

Before leaving the subject of respiratory allergies we should consider, necessarily briefly, as it is a complex subject, allergic colds and sinus troubles. In my experience, air pollution is the most common cause of chronic colds and sinus trouble in large cities in this country. I'm impressed with the lower incidence of these illnesses among persons who live at a distance from the cities. Every autumn I see the sad parade of children in my New York City office, with their runny noses, dripping sinuses, hoarseness and croupy coughs. By and large these had been healthy kids all summer at camp out of town. One of my patients, Bradford G., an 8-year old boy, even started to cough and sneeze as he stepped off the plane in September at Kennedy airport, after spending a cold-free summer in Switzerland and the Riviera.

One of the major ingredients of polluted air is sulfur dioxide. Combined with water vapor this forms sulfurous and sulfuric acids. Sulfurous acid in homeopathic dilution has been one of our great specific treatment for air pollution.

Aside from air pollution as a cause of allergic colds and sinus trouble, often I have found them to result from food allergies—in particular milk allergies. One of the great homeopathic medicines for frequent colds and sinus trouble from milk allergy is *Tuberculinum bovinum*, a diluted form of the tuberculosis germ. This can be obtained from a homeopathic pharmacy.

How to Treat Skin Allergies Homeopathically

Allergies commonly affect the skin, particularly as eczema or hives. In my experience eczema is more common among children than adults. When present it is usually brought on by many foods, in particular milk, wheat and eggs. Since it is so hard to limit a growing child's intake of these foods—also hard on the nerves of any parent who tries to enforce such a diet—homeopathic medicines offer a desirable alternative. If the eczema is dry and itchy, particularly in the creases of the elbows and knees, and worse in the winter, better in the summer, in chilly children, then *Sepia officionalis* (the dark brown-red ink of the Squid) may give relief. Interestingly, another ocean product, the ground-up shell of the oyster *(Calcarea os-*

trearum), is useful in chilly infants with wet eczema, particularly if they are worse in general at night, with head sweats and fear of the dark.

It's interesting that medicines prepared from substances from the cold ocean would be good for chilly persons.

The other common skin allergy, hives, with its widespread involvement of the skin, accompanied by swelling, itching and pain, is called "nettle rash" in England. Anyone who has been stung by nettles can see the connection between the two illnesses. Not surprisingly, in view of the homeopathic method of medicine treatment, *Urtica urens*, the stinging nettle, in high dilution, is the most effective homeopathic medicine for hives. Its clinical effects really contain the full picture of the average case of hives—itching, swellings all over the extremities and the lips and face, accompanied by heat of the body with tingling and numbness. The nose, eyes, lips and ears may swell shut. Incidently, Urtica urens is a great medicine for gout. Following this use, the urine usually becomes profuse, dark in color and loaded with uric acid crystals, as though the body is excreting the uric acid which caused the gout in the first place. Interestingly, the nettle usually grows only near human habitation, particularly where urine and fecal matter concentrate, such as around barns, outhouses and along the borders of sewage ditches. It also grows in soils with a high salt content. When the Turkish sea rover Barbarossa (Italian for redbeard), whose real name was Khair-ed-Din, conquered Milan, he ordered salt to be spread over the ruins so that nettles might grow there. Should you wish to prepare your own dilution of nettles you can do so from the crushed plant in alcoholic tincture, one drop per nine drops of alcohol, striking this first dilution 15 times against your hand, and then proceeding, in the usual way, to the 6x and 12x dilutions.

Another medicine I have found extremely useful for hives is a high dilution of the black anemone (*Pulsatilla nigricans*) or *Pasque* (French for Easter) flower as it is called because its blossoms are frequently used in France for coloring Easter eggs. This can be prepared from the alcoholic tincture in the same manner as nettles, just described. *Pulsatilla* has hives different from those of *Urtica urens*, not as swollen and bumpy, but more superficial, with red

spots that burn and prickle "as if caused by the stings of ants."
Also, unlike the hives of *Urtica urens* which are worse from cold
water bathing, Pulsatilla hives are better from cool bathing or, indeed, coolness in any form. The *Pulsatilla* hives frequently come
from eating pork or fatty foods. The patient requiring *Pulsatilla
nigricans* is gentle, loves the fresh air and cries easily from any
provocation. It is one of the great homeopathic medicines for diseases of women, and is one, indeed, of the great homeopathic
medicines, as will be explained in more detail elsewhere in this book.
Just in passing, there is a saying in medicine that the typical gall
bladder patient is a woman, fair, fat and forty—a picture of one type
of person calling for *Pulsatilla nigricans.*

How to Treat Food Allergies Homeopathically

This use of *Pulsatilla* to relieve persons unable to tolerate pork
and fats in general is an introduction to one of the most fascinating,
and complex, areas of homeopathic usefulness for the relief of many
kinds of food allergies. As in other types of allergy treatments, you
may desensitize yourself with a medicine made of the offending
substance, or by contrast, you can take a medicine not because it is
made from the offending substance but rather, because it fits your
individual symptoms totally and thus can alter your reaction to the
offending substance. This latter method is the classic method of
homeopathic "individualization."

Of the two methods the first is easiest as all these foods are
water or alcohol soluble so that they can readily be made into dilutions in your own home in the method already described and taken
by yourself in order to see if they help. Then, if this simple method of
desensitization has not helped, you can try the classic method of
homeopathic individualization by one of the standard homeopathic
medicines. So many allergies can be helped and so many medicines
are involved in their treatment that any detailed description is not
possible within the framework of this book, and may, indeed, call for
the skilled help of a homeopathic physician. For example, an allergy
to just one food, milk, may respond to any one of 57 homeopathic

medicines. Also, viewed in another way, one medicine may help many food allergies. For example, a high dilution of the Anemone, *Pulsatilla nigricans*, is of value, in bad reactions to butter, bread, cabbage, coffee, cold food, dry food, fat, fruit, meat, milk, pancakes, pastry, pork, raw food, rich food, sauerkraut, and warm food. By "bad reactions" is meant not only one or more of the classic signs of allergy such as asthma, hay fever, hives and eczema or intestinal upsets, but also the making worse of any symptoms, such as a headache which becomes worse after eating pork, or a cough made worse by coffee. Thus, by viewing patients in the broadest possible sense as total human beings, homeopathic physicians have greatly expanded the usual concept of allergy to include many reactions of aggravation (or worsening) often overlooked.

Although we cannot make any extensive evaluation of the homeopathic medicines useful in food allergies, we can consider a few of the outstanding ones.

For example, certain commonly used foods such as Coca-Cola and other cola drinks, coffee, tea, chocolate and fermented spirits, actually contain drugs such as caffeine (in tea, coffee and coca-cola), theophylline (in tea), theobromine (in chocolate) and ethyl alcohol (in fermented spirits). Many persons have had reaction to these drugs, but, because they have become addicted to them (yes, chocolate is also addictive) they don't do the obvious and sensible thing and just discontinue them. Certain homeopathic medicines can help overcome the ill effects of the misuse of these substances. Chief among them is the poison nut, *Nux vomica*, which in high dilution can relieve bad effects of coffee, alcohol, spices or just food in general. As you may remember, Nux vomica is good for oversensitivities of many kinds—to noises, odors, lights, music—indeed to life in general, so that apparently trivial ailments are unbearable, or the slightest admonition offends, making a person angry, peevish, irritable, impatient, quarrelsome, spiteful, and, sometimes, downright malicious. One person in need of Nux vomica can make a whole family miserable. Nux vomica is also good for persons who have been made worse by cold food or drinks. For instance, stomach upsets are common in the summer after people take cold food or drinks in excess or too rapidly. *Arsenicum album*, or arsenic trioxide, is also useful for such complaints, particularly diarrhea which follows the use of cold drinks in hot weather.

Another medicine with many uses is common charcoal, or *Carbo vegetabilis*. In addition to helping the bad effects of alcoholic drinks, it is outstandingly useful for the ill effects of fat foods, in particular, pork.

Finally, accustomed as we are to thinking of milk as the most important source of calcium, it should not surprise us that calcium carbonate, in the form cf ground oyster shells, *Calcarea ostrearum*, is specific for intolerance to milk.

The Homeopathic Treatment of Environmental Allergies

This broad view of human illness and of medicine action expands our view of the causes of allergies from the usual dusts, pollens, foods, chemicals, cosmetics, etc., to the environment itself. Thus, in homeopathic treatment there are medicines for persons who are worse from open air, stuffy rooms, the hot, the cold, wet weather, dry weather, changing weather, windy weather, spring, autumn, winter, summer, bathing, tight clothing, walking, standing, sitting, lying down, tobacco smoke, the sun, the seashore, riding in a car, in motion, etc.,etc. The daytime and nighttime periods of aggravation can be just like clockwork, specific to the hour, like the moss, *Lycopodium clavatum*, which is worse at 4 p.m., or Arsenic trioxide, *Arsenicum album*, which is worse at 2 a.m. Like the food allergies, any one of these environmental and situational allergies can have 100 or more medicines which may bring relief, if indicated by a person's symptoms. These we will consider in Chapter 8.

7

Homeopathic Medicines for Childhood Ailments

As we have all been children in the past—in fact many of us "so-called adults" (to use James Thurber's apt phrase) are still children emotionally—our subject is one with which we are all familiar. Even more recently, many of us have cared for children—our own, our grandchildren or the children of others.

Why Homeopathy Is Particularly Suited for Children

For me, the homeopathic treatment of children has always been particularly satisfying. Homeopathy has such unique benefits to offer children that I always feel privileged to be an instrument for their healing. The natural, gentle effectiveness of homeopathic treatment is as if made specifically for the complex, delicate growth of children through all the varied stages between infancy and adulthood. And how better to treat a child than by a largely conversational evaluation in the friendly atmosphere of a doctor's office followed by medicines which taste like candy! What a pleasure it is for me to hear children begging for more homeopathic medicine, or vying with each other as to who is the lucky one to be treated that day! And what a comfort to the child not to be assaulted by the strange odors and painful mechanical procedures of required laboratory tests before treatment can commence! And how satisfying it is for me to be able to spare my homeopathic children the bizarre, painful, incapacitating and often permanently crippling or even fatal medicine side-reactions, which might otherwise occur, particularly among unusually sensitive or delicate children! Fathers also like homeopathic treatment of their children as visits to the doctor are cheaper (particularly the medicine bills) and operations and expensive laboratory evaluations can often be avoided! Also, there are fewer tantrums when the kids have to go to the doctor!

Homeopathic treatment does not limit itself to the treatment of one segment of children but, rather, may be useful in all the five phases of childhood: the newborn, infants, childhood, adolescence, and early adulthood. Of these five normal periods of growth, infants and the newborn probably are the most difficult for homeopathic treatment both because of their natural complexity as they adjust to their new world and because of their inability to communicate their symptoms verbally to the physician. Homeopathic treatment, as I have stressed before, depends on the physician's knowledge of the subjective complaints and reactions of a patient. However, as with the treatment of animals, in spite of this major difficulty, close observation and common sense can provide a wealth of information about the most silent patient.

Homeopathic Treatment of the Newborn

The newborn have certain conditions unique to their period. As the result of passing through the birth canal, accompanied by instrumentation by his attending physician, newborn Jimmy C. showed bruises and swelling of his head and face. These were not serious and normally disappear spontaneously within a day or so. However, since his bruises lasted for a few days he received a 6x dilution of the Leopard's Bane herb, *Arnica*, followed in one day by a 6x dilution of the Marigold, *Calendula*, which relieved him in one day. Sometimes the fontanelle (or moulded area) on the top of a newborn's head is grossly swollen and does not return to normal size within a few days. Should this occur do not be alarmed. It is not usually a serious condition and often responds to a 6x or 12x dilution of the ground oyster shell, *Calcarea ostrearum*, or to a high dilution of white sand, *Silica*.

How to Treat Hernia of the Newborn

Often, newborn children will show swellings around their navel. These swellings may vary in size from a hazel to a walnut. They often enlarge if the baby cries, coughs, sneezes or does anything which increases the abdominal pressure. These swellings are hernias and usually call for surgical correction. However, if they are small they sometimes shrink after treatment with high dilutions of the herb *Nux vomica*.

Remedies for Jaundice in the Newborn

Often, newborn children are yellow at birth (jaundiced) but this usually passes within a day or so. Should it continue beyond this period, treatment may be indicated. Of course, jaundice in the newborn may come from an Rh incompatability in the blood, usually treated with transfusions of normal blood. When jaundice is not from a vascular origin, homeopathic treatment is often helpful. Outstanding among medicines for this condition is a 6x dilution of the element *Mercurius*, or often, a high dilution of the herb quinine, *Cinchona*. These are both chilly medicines but the person needing Cinchona often has a shaking chill like the malaria for which Cinchona (or quinine) is a specific. Also, Cinchona is a gassy remedy, as great as charcoal, *Carbo vegetabilis*, with gas expelled both by the mouth and the rectum, accompanied by profuse perspiration. *Mercurius* also has it discharges, in the form of excessive salivation and foul perspiration. As *Mercurius* is poisonous in gross dosage, rather than making your own you had best get a 6x or 12x dilution from the homeopathic pharmacy.

Remedies for Eye Inflammation of the Newborn

Gonorrheal infection of the eyes in the newborn still occurs at times. This condition is less common in modern times, though, because of the routine use of silver nitrate or antibiotics to prevent it.

Sometimes eye trouble appears as an inflammation from silver nitrate. Therefore it is wise to begin treatment with the homeopathic version of silver nitrate, *Argentum mitricum*, in high dilution, which may often give relief. If this doesn't help, try a 6x dilution of Monkshood, *Aconitum mapellus*. If the child is worse on waking but improves after waking, and is also worse from cold and damp, a dilution of *Rhus toxicodendron*, the poison ivy, may be indicated.

How to Treat "Red Gum" in the Newborn

Another common complaint of newborn infants is what is called "red gum," a rash of red pimples, combined with red patches about the face, neck and hands. It usually passes in a few days and is not serious. However, if it should last for more than a few days, or if it should disappear and then reappear, a little of the Leopard's Bane, *Arnica*, will often relieve it or, if that doesn't do the trick, some antimony sulfide, *Antimonium crudum* 6x, possibly followed by a 12x of the squid, *Sepia*. If the child is considerably fretful and irritated a dilution of Monkshood, *Aconitum*, may be indicated.

How to Treat Swollen Breasts in the Newborn

Finally, most newborn children of either sex have swollen breasts, a mild condition which soon passes if the breasts are left alone. Unfortunately nurses, or sometimes mothers, will squeeze the breasts to encourage a discharge. Far from helping the child, this just complicates matters. If it has been done to the child a dilution of Arnica is indicated or, if pus has formed, a 12x of sulphuret of lime, *Hepar sulph*, is best obtained from a homeopathic pharmacy.

Probably the most pressing problems for parents (or grandparents) of infants are feeding and skin problems.

How to Treat Diaper Rash

Diaper rash, as well as rashes practically anywhere else, are usually first on the scene. Humphrey N.'s rash was fiery red, worse from bathing and heat, and better in the open air, so he received a 6x of the element Sulfur which set things right in a day. On the other hand, John M. was a cold, cranky baby who perspired profusely from the head at night and was better from warmth, so he received a 12x dilution of the oyster shell, *Calcarea ostrearum* which helped his rash in 6 hours. As Dorothy M. was extremely restless and had a dry, hot skin and fever she received a 12x dilution of the Monkshood, *Aconitum*, which helped in one day. If that hadn't done the trick I would have tried the herb *Chamomilla*, which you can easily make from an alcoholic tincture of the herb, prepared in the usual manner to a 6x or 12x dilution.

Relief of Infant Colic

Colic, characterized by excessive fretfulness, crying and gas, often accompanies the rashes. Colic of this type is of unknown origin. The symptoms certainly are connected with digestion but it does not follow that food or feeding habits cause it. An old-wives' tale says it is most frequent in children superior in intellectual, emotional or physical abilities, which may give some comfort to parents afflicted with a colicky baby. In any event, it usually passes after the third month of life.

If the colic is accompanied by flatulence and vomiting and may have been caused by rich, fatty foods, a 12x of the Anemone, *Pulsatilla*, may help. If from overfeeding, in chilly irritable children, then a high dilution of the herb Nux vomica may help, or if it follows a fit of anger or exposure to the cold, a 12x of the herb Chamomilla helps. Sometimes colic can come from worms, in which case, a 12x dilution of wormwood, *Cina*, may help.

How to Treat Diarrhea in Infants

Of common occurence, diarrhea may be a sign of impending illness or simply a reaction to indigestible food. A recent patient of mine, John N., an infant of six months, suffered from slimy green, smelly stools for a few days before the mother brought him to me— naturally on a Friday at 4 p.m., just before my office was to close for the weekend. It seems to be human nature to put off seeing the doctor until the last possible minute. John's mother told me her boy was constantly fretful and ceased crying only when she held him, to recommence when she put him down in order to care for her seven other children. With his angry red face and swollen belly John looked a bit like a tomato. He was constantly moving, kept his legs drawn up against his abdomen, and passed constant slimy, greenish water stools that smelled like rotten eggs. His anus was red and raw. All this was a typical picture of a person needing the herb *Chamomilla*, one 6x powder of which immediately made a new person of John (and his mother!)

Another child in my practice, Sharon G., a little girl of four months, suffered repeated attacks of vomiting accompanied by blood-streaked, putrid smelling stools, apparently following some strange food. Sharon's face was pale and she cried constantly. A 6x dilution of the South American herb *Ipecac* soon set things alright.

Another infant, Eustice R., an eight-month old boy, developed diarrhea after a chill, accompanied by copious watery stools with a sour odor, severe colicky pains, profuse night sweats, shivering chilliness, excessive salivation, gas, small ulcers in the mouth, redness of the anus, and such straining with his stool that part of his anus actually prolapsed outside of his body. This last symptom naturally concerned the parents as they feared their boy would have to be operated upon. However, a 12x of the element *Mercurius* relieved all these problems in four hours.

Another infant, Richard O., had diarrhea with watery, slimy stools accompanied by a yellow or white coated tongue with a red tip, colic, gas, extreme fretfulness and occasional protrusion of the anus after stool. The diarrhea often alternated with constipation and the stool often contained portions of undigested food. A 12x dilution of the herb *Nux vomica* gave relief in 12 hours. Incidentally the Wild Hops, *Bryonia alba*, also is good for alternate diarrhea and constipation accompanied by undigested food in the stools, but Bryonia diarrheas may recur when the weather is warm whereas Nux vomica diarrheas are better in the warmth and worse in the cold. The homeopathic dilution of the snake venom, *Lachesis*, also relieves diarrhea alternating with constipation, particularly if the diarrhea is worse after sleeping and the stools are pale white or black and sticky.

As diarrhea is an infant's chief defense against new, disagreeable foods, the foregoing discussion of diarrhea may often apply to infants during weaning, as moving from a single, simple, healthy food like breast milk to the too many and too often unhealthy or poisoned foods we adults foolishly partake of, since this is a difficult transition for a little infant to make.

Literally, the health of future generations is in the hands of the parents, particularly the mothers of the young. If they insist that correct foods and eating habits be enforced from infancy, the great majority of later human illness can be prevented. That a large percent of disease among so-called advanced nations comes from incorrect eating habits has been shown by repeated studies of the health and eating habits of so-called primitive people. These studies all show that people eating primitive, natural, unbleached, unrefined and unprocessed whole foods have little ill health as we know it, save for infections and contagions largely brought to them by invaders from other cultures. For instance, the first travelers to the Western Hemisphere and to the Pacific were struck by the almost perfect health of the natives. However, within fifty years of colonization (a polite term for invasion) and "civilization," their health was ruined by diseases, such as smallpox and yellow fever for which they had no resistance. Even the "mild" illness of European childhood like measles killed thousands of Hawaiian natives.

Homeopathy is particularly useful in the treatment of the acute epidemic diseases of childhood, offering alternatives to the usual bed rest, supportive nutrition and the *suppression* of any secondary symptoms or infections, such as the medical suppression of the cough that sometimes accompanies measles and other infections, a suppression which often complicates or delays full recovery from the illness.

Homeopathic treatment, on the other hand, since it is directed to the person having the disease, rather than the disease which has the patient, usually lessens the severity and shortens the course of the child's illness.

How Epidemic Diseases of Childhood Respond to Homeopathic Treatment

The great homeopathic medicine for measles is *Pulsatilla*. It is useful in all stages of measles, the catarrhal (like a common cold), the eruptive (when the rash has appeared) and the convalescent (particularly when measles has been followed by inflammation of the eyes and eyelids, earache, diarrhea or discharges from the eyes or ears). Therefore, if you suspect your child is coming down with measles a 6x dilution of Pulsatilla may relieve a subsequent attack— so much so, that it is all finished in a day or so, with minor discomfort, instead of lasting the usual week or two of misery.

Some children, particularly if they are allowed to go outdoors too soon, may develop chronic conditions which could plague them the rest of their lives. For this, homeopathy offers our great medicine *Morbillinum*, made from infected measles tissue, first abstracted with ethyl alcohol, and then made into the 6x and 12x dilutions in the usual manner. Obviously you should buy this, and not make your own.

I remember an elderly lady, Mrs. Mortimer L., who came to me many years ago with an assortment of complaints. For some reason I have now forgotten, I gave her *Morbillinum*. On her next visit Mrs. C. said "Doctor, I can't believe it, but I can hear again in my left ear. It's been deaf since I had the measles as a young girl, but I got so used to it I didn't even mention it to you!"

This use of a disease product to treat the bad effects of previous diseases is one of the great contributions of homeopathy. Unfortunately this method is still unique to homeopathy, as the non-homeopathic physicians have not yet put it into general use as they did the homeopathic use of high dilutions of disease substances to *prevent* subsequent disease. I have seen hundreds of seeming miracles accomplished through the years by means of this use of disease substances to heal the bad effects of previous disease.

If however, *Morbillinum* does not help the diarrhea which may follow measles try a high dilution of the oyster shell, *Calcarea ostrearum* or, again, *Pulsatilla*. For running of the ear after measles try a dilution of the element Sulfur. For inflammation of the glands in front of and below the ear try a 6x dilution of the Leopard's Bane, *Arnica*, or the herb, Bittersweet, *Dulcamara*, both of which you can make from the alcoholic tinctures should you care to do so. If the skin is tender try a 12x dilution of the poison ivy, *Rhus toxicodendron*.

Chicken pox is usually of shorter duration than measles and less often leaves complications. For the initial fever a 6x dilution of the Monkshood, *Aconitum*, is often useful or if there is great restlessness and anxiety, a high dilution of ordinary coffee, *Coffea*. When the vesicles have formed, a 6x dilution of *Antimonium tart*, tartar emetic is useful. For complications after chicken pox try its disease product, *Variola*, in high dilution.

Like chicken pox, if uncomplicated the disease of mumps lasts only a few days. For the initial fever and swelling of the face I find nightshade, *Belladonna*, and the element *Mercurius* to be most effective, or if there is great fever and restlessness, *Aconitum*. If the testicles become affected Pulsatilla is useful. For complications after the mumps, it's homeopathic form, *Parotidinum*, in high dilutions is highly effective. If given at the onset of mumps it often moderates its course.

Whooping cough (spelled "Hooping" cough in the middle 1800's) is usually not serious in children over the age of one. This disease, however, is a terrible nuisance to other members of the family as the characteristic seal-like cough may last day and night for weeks or even months, making rest impossible for everyone. This is particularly trying as whooping cough usually hits a community in January, when we particularly need our rest to keep up our resistance.

In the early feverish and mucousy stage of the illness, before the characteristic cough has become established, further development of symptoms may sometimes be prevented.

When there is much fever and thirst, a hot skin and a rapid pulse, with a dry, frequent cough and redness and sensitivity of the eyes, then a 6x dilution of the Monkshood, *Aconitum*, may help. If the child is worse at night with restlessness, crying, a dry skin and a hollow, barking cough which is followed by violent sneezing, try the Nightshade, *Belladonna*, in high dilutions.

Scarlet fever is usually treated nowadays with antibiotics, followed by prophylactic penicillin throughout childhood to prevent Rheumatic Fever. For this reason I shall mention just a few of the outstanding scarlet fever medications.

The outstanding medication, both as a preventative during epidemics and as a cure, is a high dilution of *Belladonna*. If this does not relieve—particularly if the child develops profuse salivation, sore gums, an offensive breath, swelling of the glands of the neck and chills and shivering alternating with fever—give the element Mercurius in high dilution.

How Skin Conditions, Bedwetting and Teething Respond to Homeopathy

Ringworm is a common nuisance of childhood, often running through families. It usually responds to high dilutions of the squid, *Sepia*, followed by the poison ivy, *Rhus tox*, or the element, *Sulfur*, if needed. When it returns each year, the alternate use of Sepia and Sulfur at intervals of a week may help prevent its recurrence.

At about the time the teeth first come in, children frequently develop numerous small, white pustules on a reddish base. These usually first appear on the forehead and cheeks but they may spread over the entire body. This condition is called "Milk-Crust."

Usually the best medicine to start with for this condition is a high dilution of the Monkshood, *Aconitum*, particularly when the child is excitable and restless, and the skin around the affected area is red, inflammed and itching. If this relieves but does not cure, and if the irritation is worse at night and the urine has a strong, offensive odor, use a 6x of *Viola tricolor*, the common violet, or if the scalp is particularly affected and full of crusts which appear to itch excessively, then use the poison ivy, a 6x dilution of *Rhus toxicodendron*, in its place. If Rhus doesn't complete the job and if the eruption is dry, follow with a 12x of the oyster shell, *Calcarea ostrearum*, or if oozing, the Wolf's Foot, *Lycopodium*, or if the eyebrows are particularly involved, the element Sulfur. If the crust oozes a discharge which produces new crusts in unaffected areas of the skin, use a 6x dilution of the Daphne plant, *Mezereum*.

Another common ailment of children is chafing. For this, a high dilution of the herb, *Chamomilla*, often followed by Leopard's Bane, *Arnica*, usually does the trick, or if it has spread over large areas of the body, the element *Mercurius*, in high dilution, followed by

Wolf's Foot, *Lycopodium*. If none of these help, try a 6x dilution of the element Sulfur.

For styes *Pulsatilla* 6x is almost specific or if of frequent recurrence, the herb Stavesacre, *Staphysagria*, in a 12x dilution.

For prickly heat first try high dilutions of Monkshood, *Aconitum*, following with the herb, *Chamomilla*, if necessary or Wild Hop, *Bryonia*, if the eruption is suppressed, or the element Sulfur if it tends to recur frequently.

The common herb, *Chamomilla*, is the great specific for teething itself, or for any complaints such as diarrhea, rashes, colds, etc., which appear to have been brought on by teething. For some reason, mothers in this country don't use chamomile tea to any extent. In Europe, particularly on the Continent in France and Germany, chamomile tea seems to be used for fretful children as often as we in this country use aspirin for headaches. If that hasn't done the trick ordinary coffee, *Coffea*, in high dilution may help followed by the Monkshood, *Aconitum*, if necessary.

If diarrhea continues unchecked after *Chamomilla* follow with a 6x dilution of the element, *Mercurius*, or Sulfur if mercurius has not helped. If there is great heat and pulsation around the head with restlessness and sudden jerks and crying out during sleep, then the Nightshade, *Belladonna*, in 12x dilution may be useful.

Finally, bedwetting is often helped by the squid, *Sepia*, in high dilution followed, if unrelieved, by a 6x dilution of sand, *Silica*, or if the child shows evidence of worms in the stool or constantly picks its nose, Wormwood, *Cina*, in high dilution.

How Adolescent Illnesses Respond to Homeopathy

Adolescence is a trying time for both child and parent. It is also a challenge, as it sets the emotional basis for the adult emerging (hopefully!) out of each adolescent. Physically, adolescent girls may have many, varied troubles. These are discussed in the chapter dealing with the diseases of women. Other than these specifically female problems, adolescent boys and girls share, largely, facial acne. I'm sorry to say that I haven't found homeopathy of any spectacular success in the treatment of acne. Acne in girls will sometimes respond to high dilutions of the squid, *Sepia* or of calcium sulfide, *Hepar sulf.* Boys run more toward the element Sulfur. Since the Eskimo adolescents in the Arctic only develop acne after they adopt American eating habits I feel acne may be more a nutritional than a medical problem.

I find homeopathy of greatest value among adolescents for the medley of psychological problems which they suffer. The hot, restless, irritable boy who disturbed his class and whose grades were far below the level of his abilities straightened out in one week after a 12x of the element Sulfur. Marcia M., a chilly, depressed girl who couldn't function at home or at school the week before her period became more her normal self after a 12x of the squid, *Sepia*. Armand U. who panicked before each test in school, and was chilly and shy and constantly tired, immediately benefited from a 12x of sand, *Silica*. If Armand had been gassy after each meal, worse at 4 p.m. and afraid of being alone, I would have given him a 12x dilution of the Wolf's Foot, *Lycopodium*. Humphrey F. was mentally worn out from too much school work and nervous about going out in public. A 12x dilution of silver nitrate, *Argentum nitricum*, gave relief. Rolf P., a 12 year old boy, was completely indifferent to everything and weepy and homesick. Phosphoric acid, 12x, relieved him in one week. Virgil O. was too sensitive to everything—to light, noise, odors, touch, etc.—and constantly fidgety, with blue circles around the eyes and a longing for cold food and drinks. A 6x dilution of the element Phosphorus helped. The herb, *Nux vomica*, might also have been given if the sensitivity had been accompanied by gas in a quarrelsome, irritable intellectual boy who didn't go outdoors enough.

If you can obtain them, most of these medicines which are herbs can be prepared from alcoholic tinctures as previously described. The solid elements, like Sulfur and Silica, are best obtained from a homeopathic pharmacist. For teenagers, as well as others, care should be taken not to treat conditions that call for serious medical attention.

8

Homeopathic Treatment for Environmental Health Problems

Why We All Have Individual Reactions to Our Environment

We have all known people, who, although not really sick, react to their environments in a manner which makes life difficult for them as well as others. For example, my aunt Phyllis was so chilly that she kept her house at 85 degrees fahrenheit all winter. To make matters worse, she was so sensitive to drafts she couldn't stand an open window or door. In fact, Aunt Phyllis's reaction to drafts was so great that she could sense an open window or door from four rooms away.

Naturally, such being the wonders of love, my uncle couldn't stand hot, stuffy rooms and he suffered throughout every winter of his married life. Whenever he turned the thermostat down or opened a window my aunt would catch cold. Now, Aunt Phyllis wasn't sick and she would have indignantly denied that there was anything wrong with *her*, quite the contrary, as it was *other* people who had peculiar reactions to heat and cold.

Another example of unusual individual reactions is a patient of mine, Mrs. Ruth B., who always gets sick when the weather is clear and fine and is much better when it is humid, preferably raining. Her husband—you guessed it!—has arthritis which is just the opposite, worse in wet and better in clear, dry weather. All this made vacations almost impossible for them to plan. They usually had to compromise on a place of moderate humidity where neither feels particularly well but where at least neither is sick. After Mrs. B. received *Causticum* 12x, and her husband *Rhus toxicodention* 6x, their individual sensitivity was better so that they could try some new vacation spots.

There is a whole list of different individual reactions to the environment which can make for problems of one sort or another. None of them necessarily indicate disease, but they can be mighty hard to live with!

How Homeopathy Can Help Individuals Change

Because homeopathic practice is so strongly oriented toward these subtle, *individual* subjective medicine reactions, it has a unique ability to help persons with severe, unusual and disturbing reactions to their environment, an outstanding example of how homeopathy focuses on the *person* who is sick rather than the sickness alone.

Using Individual Symptoms As a Guide
Toward Treating All Your Troubles

And homeopathy doesn't stop just with helping the individual symptom that troubles you—like the excessive reaction to hot and cold. It can go on and help any other illness that bothers you. Thus, when you take a homeopathic medicine you are like a machine gunner who, with one squeeze of the trigger, can hit many targets almost simultaneously. Therefore, in this chapter when I describe a few of the outstanding homeopathic medicines for various environmental oversensitivities, I'm also describing substances that may relieve all kinds of your illnesses, be they physical, emotional or mental.

I've already discussed persons with unusual reactions to cold. There is a comparable group of persons with abnormal reactions to heat. I have called these two groups of persons the Thermostats. For each of these thermostats there is a comparable group of homeopathic medicines which may give them relief. Of the 2,000 or more medicines in the homeopathic *Materia Medica* tl e majority do have strong hot or cold reactions, so strong, in fact, that many homeopathic physicians use a patient's reactions to hot or cold to rule in or rule out whole groups of possible remedies. Obviously in these few pages we can consider only a few of all these many remedies for hot and cold people, as well as in our following discussion of other homeopathic medicine personalities such as the Window Raisers, the Barometers, the Windflowers, the Four Seasons types, the Sensitives, and others.

Remedies for the "Thermostats"

Three of the "hottest" medicines in the homeopathic *Materia Medica* are high dilutions of two elements, iodine and sulfur, and the lovely flower, the black anemone, or *Pulsatilla nigercans*. In my experience, of the three sulfur is the hottest. I think of it as the man's remedy—for the male of the house who wants the doors and windows open, likes cold drinks and sweets, is physically restless and constantly on the go, who can't tolerate standing in one place (for him shopping is torture!), who uses few covers on the bed even in the winter and sticks his feet out from them because they burn. These gentlemen often can't stand the heat and head for the shade as soon as they are in the sun. Boys needing sulfur are often extreme examples of the type. Incidentally, sulfur patients don't care for bathing and even when they do bathe they seem to attract dirt like magnets. I'm sure Huck Finn needed sulfur, as did Tom Sawyer.

There are sulfur ladies of course but they're less common.

Iodum, in my practice, has most frequently been for hot ladies. As we all know, iodine is part of the hormone secreted by the thyroid gland, and these iodine ladies present a typical picture of overactive thyroids. In addition to excessive personal warmth and aggravation from warmth, they are constantly hungry but nevertheless losing weight. They're tired scarecrows, profoundly weak and short of breath on slight exertion, accompanied by palpitations of the heart.

The other hot medicine, *Pulsatilla*, is also a woman's remedy. Indeed, it is called "the woman's remedy" as it is particularly suited to affectionate, mild, gentle, timid persons who are easily moved to laughter or tears. Also, their symptoms constantly change both in nature and position. They are as miserable in a warm stuffy room as are people requiring Sulfur, and whatever their complaints they are usually better in the fresh air. They have a dry mouth but are nevertheless thirstless, and they are worse from eating fatty or greasy food.

The three medicines I most frequently use for chilly persons are high dilutions of the ink from the squid, *Sepia officinalis*, quartz, or *Silicea*, and tissue infected by scabies, or *Psorinum*. These are all cold people, cold even in the summertime, particularly *Psorinum*. One of my patients, Mrs. C., a housewife in her fifties, wore a fur coat even in August. Other than chilliness, she was sad, certain that she was fatally ill, and also full of thoughts about ending her own life. She looked pale and sickly and told me, with great embarassment, that however often she bathed, her body had a filthy smell like decayed flesh, an odor also true of the diarrhea she had suffered from for the past few months. All these symptoms of hers were dramatic indications for *Psorinum*, a 12x dilution, which I am happy to say made a new woman of her in three months.

Psorinum is a rich remedy, full of too many characteristics to repeat here. One of its outstanding indications is for acute asthma that is *better on lying down*. Most asthma attacks are worse lying down! Psorinum is best obtained from a homeopathic pharmacy as it is a complex bacteriological product not available for your home preparation.

If your feet are ice cold all the time, so that you have to wear bed socks even in temperate weather, the chances are you need a little quartz sand, or Silicea! This is particularly true if you tend to catch cold if your feet become chilled. Silicea-needing persons are cold all the time, even when exercising. Although the chilliness is not as extreme as that of Psorinum, it is like it in containing a great variety of symptoms, too numerous to include here. However, a thumbnail sketch should be adequate for home treatment purposes.

Silicea people lack sand, the substance itself. They tend to sit back, have no "git up and go." They easily become overtired from slight physical or mental exertion. They are also weak emotionally, tending to be passive and introverted. Even their body processes are weak. Any little skin injury becomes infected. The muscles are weak and the digestion poor. The nails are twisted and poorly developed.

They tend to leave things unfinished, even when practically completed. Many of the school drop-outs could do with a dose of silicea. Yet, in spite of this tendency not to finish things, they can be head strong and obstinate about having their own way.

As all of us know, sand is not soluble in water or alcohol: therefore, you had better not try to prepare your own dilutions of it, but, instead, get them from a homeopathic pharmacy.

Sepia is as chilly as Silicea, but more chilly all over, where Silicea feels the cold particularly in the feet. As I have mentioned before, Sepia in high dilution is the great medicine for women's troubles of all kinds, in all stages of their lives, at the beginning, during, or at the end of their menses or from pregnancy and childbirth. Women who need Sepia usually show great sadness and weeping combined with a ready irritability and indolence. The face often has a sallow, greasy look to it and the hair looks dull and stringy and falls out in bunches.

Remedies for the "Window-Raisers"

Related to the Thermostats are the Window Raisers, crazy for fresh air. Understandably, persons needing hot remedies like the anemone, *Pulsatilla*, and the chemicals, Sulfur and Iodum, would also be fresh air fiends. To their symptoms you can add that of window raising and door opening. By contrast with the Hot Remedies, some of the most cold remedies are also Window Raisers. In particular this is true of vegetable charcoal, *Carbo vegetablis*. Persons needing high dilutions of this remedy have such a need for fresh air that they are better off no matter whatever bothers them if they are just fanned! Although basically chilly, they are worse from being overheated. As I mentioned about this remedy in the section on intestinal problems, it helps for intestinal gas of all types, as well as for troubles following too much fatty food.

Coincidentally, people needing another medicine for gas, the clubmoss Wolf's Foot, (or *Lycopodium clavatum*) also feel better in the fresh air. Maybe they need fresh air to get rid of all that gas!

Lycopodium, as you probably remember from the previous section on intestinal problems, is a predominantly right sided medication. Persons needing high dilutions of it are worry-warts, hate being alone, and are unsure of themselves, particularly before stressful situations like examinations or public appearances. They tend to be worse from 4-8 p.m.

Remedies for the "Barometers"

Related to the Thermometers and the Window-Raisers, are the Barometers, who can sense every change in the weather. Probably you know persons who can tell whenever it is going to rain, or to clear up. Commonly, persons with bone troubles such as arthritis can do this.

Certain medicines are specific for the Barometers, in particular two flowers, *Rhododendron*, and the bittersweet,*Dulcamara*, and third, a medicine made from the tuberculosis bacillus, *Tuberculinum bovinum*. The two flower medicines you can make from your own garden, starting with the alcoholic tincture as we already described. Tuberculinum you will have to purchase from a homeopathic pharmacy.

Of the two flower remedies, Rhododendron has the greatest reaction to changing weather. Persons needing this remedy actually dread storms. They fear thunder and are worse before a storm, particularly electrical storms. It is good for bony problems such as toothache, arthritis, rheumatism and gout when these conditions are worse in changing, windy and stormy weather.

Bittersweet, by contrast, affects more the skin than the bones although it is useful in some cases of acute rheumatism. All these things follow sudden changes in the weather, particularly cold, damp and rainy weather or after exposure to damp, cold places, such as unheated basements or milk dairies.

The other Barometer medicine, Tuberculinum, is extremely broad acting, affecting many organ systems of the body. Whatever the area affected, the complaints are worse from changing weather. In my own practice, whenever a person is not doing as well as I hoped for on what seemed to me the indicated medicine, and where there is a history of tuberculosis in the family, then I find a dose of Tuberculinum may set things right, often many symptoms at once. Also, the medicines I gave ineffectively before Tuberculinum suddenly start to work properly.

In addition, I find Tuberculinum is almost specific for persons who get one cold after another, seeming to catch cold from each breath of fresh air; it is also effective for eczema spreauing over the entire body, consisting of white, bran-like scales that itch intensely, particularly at night while undressing, associated with an oozing behind the ears, in the hair and in the folds of the skin.

Remedies for the "Windflowers"

Related to the Barometers are the Windflowers, persons who are worse in the wind. The two high dilutions I use most frequently for this are the black anemone, *Pulsatilla nigercans*, and the sea squid, *Sepia officinalis*. The anemone is useful for persons whose complaints are worse from winds of any type. The squid, by contrast, is specific for those persons, often women, who are worse from *cold* winds. The ears are particularly affected. I have known countless women who complained of pain, deep in their ears, in the cold wind. Or they may complain of being chilled to the bone after exposure to the cold wind.

Both Sepia and Pulsatilla have been described, and their descriptions may be referred to elsewhere, should you wish to do so.

Remedies for the "Four Seasons Types"

Another group of homeopathic personalities related to the Windflowers and the Barometers are the Four Seasons Types, named from the changes many persons undergo at a particular time of the year. Although it is understandable that arthritis or chronic lung problems would be worse in the cold winter, and that heart attacks, strokes, high blood pressure and overweight conditions would be worse in the hot summer months, it is less understandable that stomach ulcers are often worse in the spring. Nevertheless, such is the case. In homeopathic practice there are literally dozens of medicines for those who are consistently worse at one of the four seasons. However, in my own practice certain of these medicines are most frequently used.

Certainly, for complaints from summer heat I think first of sulfur. This has been so thoroughly described in this book as to require no repetition. Another high dilution for persons worse in hot weather is potassium bichromate, or *Kali bichromicum.* This is particularly useful for gastric complaints, such as the bad effects of too much beer on a hot summer day. It's also my best medicine for mucus conditions such as sinus trouble or coughs where the mucus is tough and stringy and sticks to the parts so it is drawn into long strings. The cough is often croupy, particularly in chubby, shortnecked children. Or there may be a discharge of big plugs or clinkers from the nose.

The Winter remedies I think of are the squid, or *Sepia,* quartz, or *Silicea,* and the Poison Ivy, or *Rhus toxicodendron.* If you are chilly and develop painful cracks along the sides of your fingers each winter, then you probably need *Sepia.* If every winter you're miserable with the cold and your feet are so cold you have to wear bed socks at night, then you probably need *Silicea.* If you have arthritis that is worse in the winter, particularly in wet, snowy weather, worse on first arising in the morning but better as you move around, often accompanied by great physical restlessness and tossing around, then a pinch of poison ivy, *Rhus toxicodendron,* may set you right.

Remedies for the "Sensitives"

Just as we may be sensitive to the seasons, so we may be sensitive to environmental things such as light, sound, odors or clothing. One medicine, the poison nut, *Nux vomica,* in high dilution may help all these sensitivities. It is also specific for the bad effects of stimulants such as coffee, alcohol and tobacco smoke. Many is the husband who has blessed me for removing his wife's hypersensitivity to tobacco smoke! Nux vomica patients are often irritable and quarrelsome, full of gas and digestive complaints. There may be constant nausea after eating, particularly in the morning (this is great for pregnant ladies!). The stomach feels squeezed and heavy "as if a stone sits on it!" These persons are usually constipated, although this may alternate with diarrhea. They are extremely cold, as cold as persons requiring Sepia or Silicea.

Another extremely sensitive medicine is the element, *Phosphorus.* Persons needing this medicine are as sensitive as those needing Nux vomica, but much more delicate in nature. In contrast to Nux vomica which is useful in dark, ardent, quarrelsome types, the Phosphorus patient is usually tall and fair skinned with blonde or red hair. When young these are often the "angel children" with clear fair skins, beautiful faces and golden hair, who look too good to be in this world. Persons needing Phosphorus are weak and fidgety, complain of burning pains, and desire cold food and drinks. It's one of my best remedies to clear up old coughs, particularly when the cough is worse on going from warm to cold air and worse from laughing, talking, reading, drinking, eating or being on the left side. Phosphorus treats a peculiar aggravation by, and fear of, thunderstorms. Mrs. Lincoln was so fearful of thunder that the President had to leave his office in the White House to comfort her. Her sensitivities, her anxieties and her later insanity might all have been altered with a dose of Phosphorus.

Remedies for the "Nudists"

The Nudists are a group of persons sensitive to clothing. On a house visit many years ago, I found that Mrs. W., a woman in her 50's, had no clothes on because she couldn't stand the touch of clothing on her body. As she never stopped talking, was in her menopause, and had hot flashes—all signs for high dilutions of the venom of the Surukuku snake, *Lachesis trigonocephalis*—I gave Mrs. W. a pinch of the 12x dilution. Within one day she was able to wear a few light clothes. Another South American snake venom, from a Brazilian rattlesnake, *Crotalus cascavella*, is also outstanding for this symptom of allergy to clothing of all kinds. It's interesting that all the snakes shed their skins!

Remedies for the "Owls" and the "Chickadees"

Another way we relate to our environment is through time by the alternation of day and night as well as the passage of years. Women are particularly aware of the monthly cycle through their menses. Our feeling of awareness and our ability to think and feel and just move also respond to seasonal and daily cycles, although we may not be so conscious of this. For instance, young children—particularly boys—tend to pop out of bed raring to go. Adolescents often like to stay in bed longer. Women like to stay up late and to sleep late in the morning. Men, by and large, tend to go to bed and to get up early. Within these fairly consistent reaction patterns of us females and males, many of us have different, individual reactions. Some of us are owls, bright and alert all night and grumpy and miserable in the morning; others of us are chickadees, just the opposite. In homeopathy we have medicines for both groups—medicines which can level out the extremes of each group so the Owls are a little more cheerful in the morning, and the Chickadees can stay up to midnight occasionally without feeling miserable the next day.

For the Owls I recommend high dilutions of the Surukuku snake, *Lachesis trigonocephalis*, and the herbs Stavesacre (*Staphisagria*) and poison nut (*Nux vomica*). Of the three, Lachesis is particularly indicated. Whatever is wrong with a Lachesis patient is always worse *after* sleep. Mrs. O., one of my patients who also had the other characteristics of Lachesis—constant talking, acute sensitivity of the skin, left sidedness, and feelings of hot flashes and burning—upset her whole family's routine as she was unable to get up before 10 a.m. Or at least, if she did, she dragged around in a half-daze so she might as well have stayed in bed. As a result, her husband had to get breakfast and take care of the children. In one week, a dose of Lachesis 12x restored Mrs. O. to a more normal way of functioning, much to her family's relief.

Those needing Nux vomica have a problem different than that of Lachesis. They can't help falling asleep early in the evening, awaking at 3 or 4 a.m., then falling asleep at daybreak from which they can't be aroused. As a result they feel tired and weak all day. With this of course goes the irritability, gassiness, hypersensitivity, constipation and other symptoms of Nux vomica which I have discussed elsewhere.

By contrast, people needing Staphisagria lie awake all night and then are sleepy and grumpy in the daytime. Its other characteristics have been discussed elsewhere.

Staphisagria is good for "bride's cystitis" that urinary inflammation and burning which can follow the too constant and enthusiastic pursuit of conjugal pleasures, literally keeping the person up all night.

At the other end of the time pattern are the Chickadees, so sleepy that they collapse early in the evening, much to the distress of their families. Frequently these are husbands like Bill G.—often commuting husbands under pressure of their early morning trains.

Although early to bed and early to rise is said to make a man healthy, wealthy and wise, it also made Bill's family life difficult, particularly as he was absent all day at work. Therefore, sometimes it's desirable to moderate this pattern a bit for the sake of the other members of the family. A pinch of Sulfur 12x helped change Bill in that direction within two months.

Remedies for the "Clock Watchers" and the "Calendars"

In addition to morning and evening some of us are consistently worse or better at other times of the day. As I mentioned earlier, persons needing arsenic trioxide, *Arsenicum album*, are characteristically worse after midnight and particularly at 2 a.m. With this goes the Arsenicum picture of chilliness, restlessness, great prostration, burning pains, and so on, which have already been described. The Wolf's Foot, *Lycopodium clavatum*, is worse at 4 p.m., again accompanied by the gassiness, anxiety, irritability, etc. of Lycopodium. Some medicines are worse at wider than daily intervals. Cinchona, or quinine, has attacks, particularly of fever, which return every seven to 14 days. Ordinary clay, or *Alumina*, also is worse every 14 days often falling on either the full or the new moon. Persons needing Alumina are dry, thin, chilly and usually constipated, often accompanied by an appetite for peculiar things such as starch, chalk, charcoal, cloves, or coffee and tea grounds.

Another medicine with a clock-like periodicity is Cedron, or *Simaba cedron*, the seeds of a Caribbean and South American fruit tree first discovered by the Buccaneers. This has the unusual symptom of the repetition of any problem at the same time each day—so you can set your clock by it. Jonathan W., whose headaches returned every day at 10 a.m., lost them in two days after a 12x dilution of Cedron.

As our time reactions can be used to understand the homeopathic *Materia Medica*, equally our body reactions can illuminate another group of medications.

Remedies for the "Rights"

Just as the reactions to hot and cold, as used by a homeopathic physician, are an unusual and basically fascinating way of thinking about types of persons, so also, to a homeopathic physician, the observation that some persons have all their troubles on one side of the body provides a most useful way of discriminating between ill persons and medicine reactions. How often have you heard someone say, "I don't know why, but when I'm sick its always on one side." This can be a life long pattern. I've had patients who practically never had troubles except on one side of themselves. When they had mumps it was on that side; headaches would be one-sided; colds and flu, etc.; even accidents would be one-sided.

Put together with other groups of patient reactions such as those to hot and cold, type of weather, or time of day, these body reactions of predominant right- and left-sidedness help us discriminate between the two thousand or so medicines available for homeopathic uses.

Among the dozen or so predominantly right-sided medicines, as I have mentioned earlier in this book, the one I use most frequently is the club moss, *Lycopodium clavatum*, in high dilutions. Particularly when combined with those other characteristics of Lycopodium, such as gassiness, 4 p.m. aggravation, irritability and worrisomeness, this one-sided reaction can usually be trusted as an indication for Lycopodium. In fact, so often do I find it to hold true that, regardless of a person's basic problem, if it is predominantly right-sided, the first remedy I think of is Lycopodium. And it's amazing how often it helps.

Remedies for the "Lefts"

The left-sided medicines I use most frequently are high dilutions of the squid, *Sepia officinalis*, and the venom of the Surukuku snake, *Lachesis trigonacephalus*. Sepia is for the chilly ladies and Lachesis for the warm ones. They're both outstanding for menopausal symptoms, particularly hot flashes. The symptom pictures of both of these medicines are described elsewhere.

Remedies for the "Indians" and the "Palefaces"

Other body types I frequently see in my practice are the "Indians" and the "Palefaces." Often I can see the medicine a person needs before I have spoken a word with him. If he has a red face and is wearing lighter clothing than average in the winter he probably needs a high dilution of Sulfur, or if he has a red face and his chief complaint is a throbbing headache, a 12x dilution of nitroglycerine, or *Glonoine*, will help. If the face is extremely pale, and the person takes cold constantly, for no apparent reason, and complains of skin troubles or headaches in particular, then a dose of *Tuberculinum bovinum* 12x is probably indicated. If the pale face is in a chilly, plump person whose head sweats at night, then a high dilution of the oyster shell, *Calcarea ostrearum*, may be indicated. Or if in oversensitive persons who desire cold drinks and complain of burning symptoms scattered around the body, then a dilution of the element Phosphorus may help.

Remedies for the "Sweets Freaks"

The Sweets Freaks run to three medicines in particular: in descending order of use in my own practice, the element Sulfur, the club moss, *Lycopodium clavatum*, and the substance silver nitrate, or *Argentum nitricum*. The first two of these have been so thoroughly and frequently described in this book as to need no repetition. People requiring *Argentum nitricum* in addition to craving sugar, may develop diarrhea from eating sugar, often accompanied by great flatulence with belching after each meal. This is an outstanding medicine for diarrhea in infants which looks like chopped green spinach on the diaper. Persons needing *Argentum nitricum* often are thin. Their dried-up faces may make them appear old before their time.

Remedies for the "Salt Cellars" and the "Spice Merchants"

Chief among the Salt Cellars is, of course, salt, or *Natrum muriaticum*. In my own practice I find that persons needing charcoal, or *Carbo vegetabilis*, are next in order of frequency.

The Spice Merchants seem to need mostly the herb, *Nux vomica*, or quinine, *Cinchona*.

9

Homeopathic Strengtheners for Physical Weakness

In our lives we move from weakness, through weakness, to weakness again as we go from the weakness of birth to the weakness of age, through the various weaknesses that are part of our normal adult experience. Indeed, for many of us, strength is known only too briefly. Our lives center around and move outwards from physical weakness rather than physical strength. Of course, weakness is a relative term only given meaning by a comparison point. Compared to an ant we are immeasurably stronger, to an elephant immeasurably weaker. Children, of varying strengths among themselves, are weaker than adults and since they necessarily live in and are supported by the adult world, they remain in essence weak, as are many of the aged at the other end of the cycle of years.

As we are ringed around with weakness through the tissue of our lives, how fortunate that homeopathy has so many medicines for our many weaknesses!

A Strengthener for Weakness After Disease

Of all our varied weaknesses, those accompanying or following disease may be the hardest to bear. As I mentioned earlier, in addition to first introducing the use of disease bacteria to prevent or modify subsequent diseases, homeopathy also *uniquely* uses the products of disease to relieve the results of a particular infection or contagion. Thus, the long-term effects of all the common illnesses and infection can be treated homeopathically. An example is the use of homeopathic influenza virus to help persons who are weak following an attack of influenza. Also, since *any* bacteria, virus or disease product can be diluted and succussed for homeopathic use, it means that even the effects of newly discovered diseases can also be treated homeopathically, so that homeopathic medicines carry an endless potential for relieving weakness following any infection. And since they carry only the energy state of the bacteria rather than its chemical substance, they confer a self-healing potential with little danger of side reactions.

Constitutional Homeopathic Prescribing

In addition, since the weakness following an illness is, particularly nowadays, often the result of the medicine used to treat the illness rather than of the illness itself, a whole other aspect of homeopathic treatment presents itself—the use of homeopathic dilutions of non-homeopathic medicines to relieve their side effects in disease treatment. I often use homeopathic penicillin preparations for this effect. Again, because these can be prepared simply and cheaply, a truly unlimited number of homeopathic medicines can be prepared for the side effects not only of medicines already known, but also for medicines not as yet developed.

Practically, how does this work? Well, recently Henry S., a 22-year old pilot told me he had never recovered from the effects of a previous Asiatic influenza attack. Henry was constantly tired and subject to frequent illnesses of all kinds. As a result, both his professional and personal life were in a mess. One dose of the 12x dilution of Asiatic influenza virus, prepared for me by Nelson's Homeopathic Pharmacy in London, restored Henry to his pre-influenzal state within a week. In the past few years I must have treated scores of persons with similar post-influenzal problems.

Before the introduction of the anti-tubercular drugs, an unbelievable kind of tiredness and weakness accompanied tuberculosis, particularly in its healing phase. Homeopathic physicians of the time found that preparations of various *tubercle bacilli* helped relieve this lassitude and enervation. Even today, if I have a patient with great weakness and a history of previous but arrested tuberculosis I find the homeopathic *Tuberculinum* will often help. Or if a weak, sickly person has an immediate family history of many persons with tuberculosis, then *Tuberculinum* will often help.

Venereal diseases, unfortunately epidemic in this country now, also may leave people weak and tired even after their successful treatment with antibiotics. A dose of the appropriate homeopathic preparation of syphilitic tissue *(Syphilinum)*, for syphilis, or of gonorrheal tissue (*Medorrhinum*), for gonorrhea, will often bring relief. And, again, this may help persons with a long family history of syphilis or gonorrhea infections.

Weakness may follow many infectious diseases other than influenzal and venereal. Homeopathic pharmacists have prepared all these bacterial agents in diluted and energized form. To name just a sample—streptococci, pneumococci, diptheria, rabies, whooping cough (*pertussin*), measles (*morbillinum*), chicken pox (*varicella*), small pox (*variolinum*), mumps (*parotidinum*), poliomyelitis, and others. Even fungus infections, which sometimes can affect total body reactions, can be treated in this manner.

For instance, the *coccidiomycosis*, a dustborne fungus common in the Southwestern United States, produces pneumonia-like symptoms. A homeopathic preparation of this fungus can often help a person throw off the illness. Or, another example, because of the recent use of contraceptive female hormone pills many women have developed vaginal overgrowths of fungi, frequently one called *Monilia albicans*. The comparable homeopathic preparation of this fungus can often help the problem.

Treatment of Weakness After Hepatitis

Weakness following infections can also, of course, be treated in the manner of classic homeopathy, with the medicine indicated by the symptom rather than by a homeopathic preparation of the causative agent. For example, inflammation of the liver (or hepatitis) is an increasingly common illness among my patients. Partly, this is because people all over the world are constantly traveling back and forth, sharing illnesses which until recent times were limited to certain parts of the world. Infectious hepatitis is a virus-born disease readily transmitted by contaminated water, or food (particularly shellfish) or by contact among ourselves. With its yellow itching skin, dark brown urine and clay-colored stools it is a dramatic disease whose diagnosis is usually obvious. Accompanying these colorful symptoms are fever, restlessness, nausea and extreme weakness. These symptoms may last for months and from my experience with its victims the tiredness may last for years after all the other symptoms have gone. It is truly a catastrophic, disabling illness.

Happily, homeopathy is often able to help the unfortunate victims of hepatitis. I must have treated dozens just in the past five years. Sulfur in high dilutions appears to be specific for the post-hepatitis debility and fatigue. Just as one example, Malcolm S., an outstanding artist in his early thirties, came to me with a history of six months loss of work because of hepatitis he had brought back from Mexico. He presented the usual picture—a large, tender liver, yellow skin, dark urine and light stools. Fortunately, his young wife and newborn daughter had not contracted his illness. I prescribed homeopathic Sulfur in the 12x dilution. He didn't get steadily better but had ups and downs. Within a few weeks Malcolm was out of bed, no longer jaundiced and within a month he was back at work part-time. In the two year period since I last saw him he has done well.

Another recent victim, Joan S., a young singer, acquired her hepatitis in India where she had studied Indian music for a year, living with the peasants in small back-country villages. Like Mexico and other poor countries, these little villages have no sanitary water supply, so that waterborne diseases such as hepatitis and typhoid readily spread to foreigners who have not, like the local residents, built up some degree of immunity to the local plague of diseases. In addition to jaundice, Joan had ugly, weeping sores all over her feet. She was so weak she could barely move out of bed to go to the bathroom. A 12x dilution of two medicines, the greater Celandine, *Chelidonium majus*, and the Squid, *Sepia officinalis*, literally got her back on her feet. Once the jaundice and weakness had gone, I zeroed in on the disgusting-looking foot sores with other medicines. These disappeared after one month of treatment with Sulfur 12x. I haven't heard from her for six months or so which is a good sign as in medicine "no news is good news." Being a physician is like being a parent to an enormous family—you never hear from the kids unless they're in trouble and want something.

Incidentally, *Chelidonium*, in high dilution, is *the* specific medicine for the full picture of acute hepatitis—even more so than sulfur. Interestingly, it even looks like the liver—its leaves are liver-shaped and its sap, like bile, is a bright yellow.

Remedies for Weakness from Anemia

Another condition accompanied by extreme weakness is anemia, particularly in women of menstruating age. As we all know from ads on television, this condition may come from an iron deficiency, and therefore may respond to increased iron in the diet. However, a recent study in England showed that women with the symptoms of an iron deficiency anemia—symptoms such as tiredness, breathlessness, paleness, chilliness, and scanty menses— often have normal (although low normal) hemoglobin levels, and are *not* relieved by additional iron. Although many homeopathic medicines may help, of them all I have found high dilutions of *Sepia officinalis* to be the most helpful. Another useful homeopathic dilu- tion is charcoal, *Carbo vegetabilis*. In addition to fatigue, a pale face, cold extremities and cold perspiration—all signs of anemia—this medicine is good for the bad effects of any exhausting diseases, whether in the young or the old. For instance, I always think of *Carbo vegetabilis* for persons whose asthma dates from childhood measles or whooping cough, or for the bad effects of previous illness such as typhoid fever.

Treatments for Weakness After Surgery

Another too common cause of weakness today is that following surgical operations. As I mentioned earlier, the Leopard's Bane plant, *Arnica montana*, aids recovery from operations. In addition to physical weakness, often a psychological weakness or depression fol- lows surgical operations. For this, high dilution of St.John's Wort, or *Hypericum perforatum*, is helpful; it is also useful for psychological depression following shock or fright.

Relief of Weakness from Grief

Weakness can also follow psychological conditions such as grief or personal worries. We have all seen persons both physically and emotionally immobilized following the loss of a loved one or from long sustained worry or chagrin or care. These persons are listless, apathetic, uninterested in anything around them. Phosphoric acid 12x will often give them relief. If this doesn't help, the secretion from the whale from which perfume is made, *Ambergris* or *Ambra grisea*, is often helpful, particularly in thin, emaciated old persons (like Mrs. Helen W., a recent widow whose nerves had "worn out," and who sat for days weeping). As it is soluble in alcohol, Ambra Grisea can be prepared in the usual manner from the alcoholic tincture.

Another medicine for persons completely prostrated from long-concentrated grief is the St.Ignatius Bean, *Ignatia amara*, whose action was already described elsewhere. One of the chief guides to this medicine is involuntary sighing. These persons will just sigh and sigh and sigh, one after the other. Recently, a young woman, Mercedes W., on her first visit with me just sat in a chair, didn't move or show any expression, and sighed repeatedly. It turned out that Mercedes's boyfriend of many years had just jilted her. Ignatia 12x didn't bring him back but did make her better able to live with her grief.

Incidentally, Phosphoric acid 12x is also highly indicated for the weakness of old age, often accompanied by slow thinking from hardening of the arteries in the brain. Another useful medicine for the weakness of old age is a high dilution of the ordinary nutmeg, *Nux moschata*. These persons have a weakness of the memory so that thoughts vanish while talking, reading or writing, or they may use the wrong words in speech, or not recognize well known streets. They are absent-minded, unable to think and indifferent to everything. They are readily fatigued so they must lie down on the slightest exertion. Their mood swings widely from laughter one moment to tears the next. Like its near-relative Nux vomica, there is a great sensitivity to light, sounds, odors and to touch. It's outstanding symptom is overpowering drowsiness and sleepiness, which accompanies all complaints.

Another good medicine for a weak memory is a high dilution of the poison hemlock, *Conium maculatum*. There is no inclination for business or study, along with a complete indifference to everything. These persons are domineering and quarrelsome. They can't stand contradiction of any kind. They dread being alone but avoid society. It is one of our greatest medicines for vertigo, particularly when the vertigo is worse on lying down or turning in bed. Conium 12x will often help celibate old men or women, who suffer from the complaints of suppressed sexual desire.

Treatments for Weakness in Children

At the other end of the time scale is weakness in children. My most useful medicine for this is a 6x of barium carbonate, or *Baryta carbonica*. Although also useful for weakness in old men, both physical and mental, it is outstanding for children with weak memories. I have had numerous children through the years who responded so well to *Baryta carbonica* that their teachers couldn't believe it. Many of those who had been left behind in school were suddenly advanced to their own age level. These children often look dwarf-like, and are physically as well as mentally weak.

The club moss, *Lycopodium clavatum*, in high dilution, also helps weakness in old age as well as in children. However, persons needing Lycopodium, although physically weak, are usually intellectually keen. Along with these symptoms go the other characteristic Lycopodium symptoms we have already discussed at length—the gassiness, 4 p.m. aggravation, fear of being alone, right sidedness, the irritability and the weepiness.

The other medicine I find most useful for weak children—weak both physically and mentally— is pure silica, *Silicea*, in high dilution. These children are often weak because of poor nutrition—not from *lack* of food but from imperfect assimilation. They are tired kids, always wanting to lie down. Their muscles are soft and weak. They are also weak emotionally (they tend to quit if the going gets a little hard) as well as mentally, since thinking, reading and writing are all very difficult. Even their physiological processes are weak. They are constantly chilly, and any skin injury or infection heals extremely slowly if at all.

Treatments for Weakness from Menstruation

In between these extremes of the weaknesses of childhood and old age are the weaknesses of middle-age, particularly the weaknesses of women at different phases of their menses. Although these were already touched upon in previous chapter, they are important enough to bear repeating at this time.

For weakness before the menses I find common milk of magnesia, or *Magnesia carbonica*, in the 12x dilution, of greatest value. Accompanying this may be chilliness, bearing-down pains and backache—all a picture similar to the squid, *Sepia officinilas*, also commonly indicated for this premenstrual weakness. Just as magnesia is often needed to "sweeten" the stomach, frequently persons needing *Magnesia carbonia* have a sour disposition, a sour odor to the body and sour belching.

If the weakness before the menses is felt particularly in the legs, then a high dilution of the herb, *Cocculus indicus*, is useful. With this may go a severe nausea or vomiting from riding in any type of vehicle. Cocculus is one of our great medicines for seasickness of any types.

Sometimes the weakness is greatest during the menses. Mrs. St.D., was so weak during the menses that she could barely speak. Even the menses themselves were so weak that they only flowed in the morning. She was helped with a 12x of animal charcoal, or *Carbo animilas*. In addition to the menstrual weakness, a general weakness is present. The circulation is feeble and stagnant and general body heat is at a minimum. The joints are weak and easily sprained by slight exertion and the ankles turn while walking. The muscles are weak and easily strained from lifting, even small weights, accompanied by great weakness in general. The hearing is so weak that the direction from which sounds come cannot be determined.

Mrs. Josephine M., a 37-year old housewife, needed the White Hellebore, *Veratrum album*, as she had an extreme weakness during the menses, so extreme she could barely stand. She was profoundly cold, both by inner feeling and to the touch. Her skin felt icy cold to the touch and there was a cold perspiration on her forehead. There was a cold feeling in the abdomen but, in spite of the general feeling of coldness there was an unquenchable thirst for large quantities of ice cold water. On the least exertion, she fainted. There was a rapid sinking of all the vital forces with complete prostration and collapse. After a powder of 6x *Veratrum album*, Mrs. M. improved within two weeks. This is also one of the great homeopathic medicines for cholera, the first I think of for violent vomiting accompanied by profuse diarrhea.

When weakness follows the menses, then I find high dilutions of Phosphorus most frequently indicated. Persons needing this medicine have an extreme weakness of the whole body, accompanied by nervousness and trembling. They are uninterested in everything, move slowly and answer slowly if at all. They are weary of life and see everything as dismal and gloomy, particularly the future. These are enormously sensitive people, to all external impressions such as light, noise, odors and touch. People say of them that they're "too sensitive to live."

10

Solving Sexual Health Problems with Homeopathic Home Remedies

The very hormones which define our maleness and femaleness may also set men and women apart from one another, producing a host of physical and psychological problems. The overcoming of these sex-made differences provides both the challenge and the frustration of the relationship between men and women. Hopefully, the new open communication about human sexuality may help prevent much of the physical and psychological disease which often results from sexual problems. Unfortunately this new sexual liberty has also produced problems of its own such as increased venereal disease, but this will take care of itself once we have settled down to a saner balance between our past puritanism and our present sexual overconcern.

Why Sex Is a "Hex"

Like our own sexual apparatus, sexual problems come in all shapes and sizes, some of them even ante-dating puberty. Homeopathy has medicines for most of these problems, effective for many persons. Of course, one of the first problems regarding sexuality is what are the *problems* and what is *normal*! Sex is such a personal thing, and cultures vary so in its use, that there are almost as many standards for sexual behavior as there are people behaving sexually.

The courts naturally reflect this confusion of values regarding sexual acts. In some countries polygamy is lawful, in most countries it is not. Equally so with homosexuality.

Most countries, however, agree in forbidding all forms of antisocial sexuality such as rape, child molestation, exhibitionism etc.

Probably because of the many, unresolved differences toward sexual conduct practiced throughout society, the whole question of defining and treating sexual illnesses has been largely ignored by medicine until recent years. We all know of the Kinsey report of the 1950's and of the more recent work of Masters and Johnson in St. Louis in their photographic study of normal sexual behavior, as well as the earlier investigations of psychiatrists such as Sigmund Freud, Kraft-Ebbing, and many others. In spite of this lack of a common understanding about sexual behavior, at any given time there have been persons who have felt—probably for a mixture of complex physical and cultural reasons—that they had sexual problems. Homeopathic treatment of these persons is often highly successful.

The most common sexual problem men and women bring to their physicians is some type of sexual inadequacy. Among women this is usually experienced as pain on intercourse, or a lack of sexual desire both before and during intercourse. Men rarely experience pain on intercourse, but they may experience a lack of, or poorly sustained desire.

All these various conditions may be treated homeopathically although first a thorough physical evaluation should be made to rule out possible serious complications. Pain on intercourse in women, for instance, may come from structural changes of the female organs, calling for surgical, not medical treatment. Loss of sexual desire in young or middle aged persons may come from *diabetes mellitus* or from other serious degenerative diseases such as leukemia, or it may be associated with a profound psychological depression. In older persons this loss of sexual desire may result from a lowered level of sexual hormones in the blood stream. If present, these physical conditions—or others—must often be dealt with at their own level before homeopathic treatment is commenced.

Assuming these precautions have been taken, making homeopathic treatment possible, I have found two homeopathic medicines most commonly indicated for sexual deficiencies—the ocean going Squid, *Sepia officinalis* for women and the Club Moss, Wolf's foot, *Lycopodium clavatum*, for men.

Remedies for Loss of Sexuality

Sepia 12x is useful in all kinds of sexual difficulties in women. Chief among these is pain on intercourse, whatever the cause. It also helps ladies who have lost interest in intercourse. Many hundred of my patients with these complaints have been helped by Sepia through the years. One recent example, Mrs. Helen F., a retired school-teacher, because of her menopause, suffered shrinking and aging of her vagina. After one dose of Sepia 12x her husband was a happy man again. Incidentally, lady-like men who suffer a loss of sexual interest also often need Sepia.

If you need Sepia, in addition to the sexual problems you should have some of the other Sepia characteristics such as chilliness, feeling badly before your periods (if you are a menstruating woman), and probably some sadness or depression.

For men with sexual problems, a high dilution of the Club Moss, *Lycopodium clavatum*, is as successful as is Sepia for women. Clovis D., a recent patient of mine, suffered poor erections when he developed multiple sclerosis. Since his complaints were worse on the right side and in the afternoon—all Lycopodium symptoms—I gave him Lycopodium 12x which not only helped his erection problems in two weeks but his multiple sclerosis as well. Another patient, George S., had poor erections and loss of sexual desire since he developed *diabetes mellitus*. Again, Lycopodium 12x restored the erections, although not 100%, as well as helping the basic diabetic condition. Although both these men had been impotent only a few months, Lycopodium may also help impotence of many years' duration. When prescribed for impotence, Lycopodium works best if its characteristic symptoms of gas after eating, right-sided complaints, a 4 p.m. aggravation, excessive worrying and nervousness before tests or public appearances are present.

Treatments for Injured Sexuality

A number of other medicines are useful for impotence. For example, Basil Z., a young man of 28 in my practice, suffered impotence following a severe football injury to his penis. Although everything seemed well structurally, his erections were painful, resulting in an inability to retain them, a matter of great concern both to Basil and his wife. A 12x powder of the Leopard's Bane, *Arnica montana*, fixed him up in one month. Sometimes an injury to the spine—particularly to the lower spine, from which point originate the nerves which control the sexual organs—will produce sexual impotence. One of my patients, Herman H., a young man of 22, suffered this unfortunate affliction after he was thrown from his horse. Fortunately, a pinch of St. John's Wort 6x—or *Hypericum perforatum*—fixed him up in one week. All of these medicines are herbs, so you can make them yourself if you wish.

Overcoming Impotence

The great specific for impotency which is stressed by the homeopathic textbooks is the "Chaste Tree"—certainly a descriptive name!—*Agnus castus*. *Agnus castus* treats the classic picture of impotence—premature old age, melancholy, apathy, self-contempt—associated with no sexual power or desire.

A Remedy for Tired Casanovas

Finally, I have found high dilutions of Phosphoric acid most helpful for men who became impotent through sexual excesses. These persons are listless, apathetic and indifferent to life in general. As phosphoric acid is hard to find in your community, you had best obtain it from a homeopathic pharmacy.

Relief of Pain on Intercourse

We have already considered Sepia for women who have pain on intercourse. Certainly it is my most useful medicine for this condition—a condition probably responsible for more marital unhappiness in both husbands and wives than any other. Another very useful medicine for this condition is the common herb Stavestacre or *Staphisagria*. You can prepare an alcoholic tincture from the plant in your garden. This is helpful for vaginal pains so severe that just the pressure of clothing becomes intolerable. Persons needing this medicine are often extremely proud and sensitive, indignant over imagined or real wrongs, and full of unexpressed rage and hostility.

How to Treat Female Spasms

A particularly nonresponsive type of feminine pain on intercourse comes from a constriction of the sexual organs, making entry into them impossible or so painful as to be unbearable. This condition often responds to lead, or *Plumbum*, in homeopathic form.

A Remedy for Excessive Sexuality

In this day of gross oversexuality we may forget that excessive sexual activity or overconcern can be as much of a problem as impotence for men or pain on intercourse for women. Although I have had a few women patients with this complaint of excessive sexual concern mostly they seem to be males. Since this kind of sexual preoccupation seems to be normal for healthy males—in the army sex and food were the main subjects of discussion—my patients have, necessarily, been persons who felt they had a problem which needed attention. In other words, I didn't make the judgment of sexual overconcern, but the patients did.

Among men this type of preoccupation can lead to excessive masturbation, sometimes a number of times a day. Obviously, this degree of sexual preoccupation can interfere with school or work routines—even, paradoxically, marital routines, since the average woman isn't willing to submit to this type of constant intercourse. For instance, Joseph R., a man in his forties, even though he has been married for many years still masturbated a number of times a day. He felt guilty about this and had a "hangdog" expression with blue circles under his eye. Understandably Joseph was tired and apathetic in general and had difficulty coping with life. A 12x dilution of the element Phosphorus relieved him in six weeks. If this fails to help, the related medicine Phosphoric acid, which has a similar action picture, will often help. Another acid, Picric acid, has a similar sexual picture to that of Phosphoric acid. There is the same profound weariness and aggravation from any activity—physical or emotional. In addition, persons needing high dilutions of Picric acid have long-lasting, violent erections. Interestingly, the calcium salt of phosphorous, *Calcarea phosphorica*, also helps men with excessive erections, as well as women with excessive sexual preoccupation.

How to Treat Loss of Desire

Possibly you saw the secret agent movie set in Japan in which the hero, following torture, has lost his usually voracious sexual appetite. When her patience wears thin, his Japanese girlfriend goes to a local folk healer and buys from him a medicine made of excretion from a toad's skin. There's a dramatic scene in which a large and extremely ugly toad—probably the ugliest toad available—is given gentle shocks to stimulate secretion, of toad sweat. When given to the hero, this toad medicine sets thing right again.

Amusingly, this episode is based on fact, for the secretion of *Bufo rana,* the common toad, will produce sexual overstimulation in the healthy male.

Remedies for Sexy Ladies

In this day of woman's lib it would not be right to leave this subject without mentioning medicines specific for women who have excessive sexual preoccupations. The one I have found most useful in my own practice is the element platinum, or *Platina*, in high dilutions. Women needing this remedy have excessive sexual desires. Their organs are highly developed—even in virgins—and so sensitive that even the touch of clothing is unpleasant. The sensitivity may be so great as to render intercourse unbearably painful, even resulting in fainting. Along with this goes a strongly defined temperament—proud, contemptuous and haughty, alternately gay and sad. The menses are often too early and too profuse, with dark clots.

Another great medicine for overly sexy ladies is, of all things, the common garden herb sweet Marjoram, or *Origanum*. There is great sexual excitement, often driving this type of woman to daily masturbation, making her unable to carry out her daily responsibilities.

Finally, we should consider briefly the homeopathic treatment of homosexuality. Through the years I have had a few of these unfortunate persons as patients. I say unfortunate not in a patronizing sense, but because however happy and adjusted they may be to their own sexual needs, inevitably they are exposed to the often cruel judgments of society.

There are many theories—none proven—about the causes of homosexuality. According to the orthodox psychiatric view it is the result of childhood conditioning. Geneticists, in the other hand, trace it to an abnormal chromosomal pattern in the sexual development of the fetus.

Some Medicines for Homosexuality

Whatever its cause, I have found it to be an extremely difficult condition to treat homeopathically. Although many homosexuals—both men and women—have been my patients through the years, for one reason or another, only a few have asked my help in overcoming their homosexuality, and I can't honestly claim any success in that endeavor. However, one of my teachers claimed to have cured a male homosexual with repeated high doses of the element Phosphorus over a period of many years. And some other colleagues maintain they have treated women homosexuals successfully with the marine squid, *Sepia officinalis*, and also common sea salt, *Natrum muriaticum*, both in high dilutions.

SECTION II
HOMEOPATHIC MATERIA MEDICA

HOMEOPATHIC MATERIA MEDICA

Discussing homeopathic treatment in terms of *illnesses*—as we have so far—naturally produces a spotty knowledge of each medicine. Since the more you know about a given homeopathic medicine the better you can use it, in this Section II, all the different characteristics of each medicine we have considered have been gathered together.

Every medicine is listed alphabetically, by its scientific name (usually in Latin such as *Arnica montana*), the abbreviation of this scientific name such as ARN, and its most common, or everyday name in English, such as Leopard's Bane. Thus, each medicine is listed in three ways. Another example is *Natrum muraticum*, NAT-M, or common table salt.

Below its name, the characteristic symptoms of each medicine are listed alphabetically.

This grouping together of the homeopathic medicines, each with its characteristic symptoms, is called a *Materia Medica*. Just as a carpenter needs his tools in order to build a house, so, the homeopathic physician must have a knowledge of the vast homeopathic *Materia Medica*—over two thousand tested medicines, some running thousands of characteristic symptoms—in order to practice homeopathic therapy. If you become acquainted with this small, beginners' homeopathic *Materia Medica*, you will be able to help yourself and others with gentle, natural nontoxic medicines.

Even a small *Materia Medica* such as this can be difficult to remember in toto. Also, when you have once read this book, it's a nuisance to have to refer back to a particular chapter in order to find a medicine which may help. In addition, some useful treatment tips are mentioned as asides from the regular subject of a chapter, so that you would have to read the entire book in order to find them.

Since a symptom guide to the *Materia Medica* would solve these problems, it has been provided in Section III. After first evaluating your own symptoms—in particular what makes them better or worse—you can turn to the symptom guide and seek a medicine specific to your needs.

For instance, say you have arthritis, with aching pains throughout your joints, worse in cold wet weather, or after rest, and better in warm dry weather and after exercise, and now you wish to find one medicine which fits all these symptoms. If you turn to your symptom guide you will see *Rhus toxicondendron* and *Sepia* listed under "joints, pains, and heat improves." But since only Rhus tox is improved by exercise, that has to be your medicine.

As a final check you may wish to review the description of *Rhus tox* in the *Materia Medica*, just to make sure the picture fits.

If you were worse from motion, then *Calcarea ostrearum* might help you. Actually, *Calcarea ostrearum* is often needed to complete the action of Rhus tox, so if you find that *Rhus tox* gives you only temporary relief, and if you are a chilly person who has other symptoms, such as head sweats at night, then a powder of *Calcarea ostrearum* after *Rhus tox* may give you more permanent improvement.

Out of the whole conglomeration of symptoms described for a particular medicine, you may find that you have only a few. Don't let this disturb you, as long as you don't have symptoms strongly *opposed* to the medicine picture. For instance, you don't *have* to be chilly for *Calcarea ostrearum* to relieve you of other of its symptoms, but if you are a *hot* person, probably you should consider another medicine for yourself.

In addition to being highly useful, this search for the right homeopathic medicine is lots of fun!

ACON
Aconitum Napellus
Monkshood

Air, fresh, improves
Anxiety
Appetite, lost
Chicken pox, fever
Colds, after chill
  from exposure to cold
Cough, dry
  frequent
  from cold winds
  from drafts
  from dry winds
  short
Diaper Rash, in
     restless, feverish
     babies
Eyes, inflammation
  inflammation in newborn
  redness of
  sensitivity of
  tearing
Face, eruption,
     pustules at teething
  eruption, red, patches in
     newborn
  red
  red and pale alternate

Fear, death
  seasickness
Fever
Head, pressing
    outwards sensation
  top of, warmth of
Immobile
Kidney disease
Leg, swollen, watery, hot
  swollen, watery, painful
Measles, fever
Menses, absent due to chill
  suppressed from being chilled
  unendurable pains with
Mind, dullness of
Mouth, dry
Nose, running
Pulse, rapid
Respiration, fast
  hot
Restless
Restlessness, emotional
  physical
Skin, dry
  hot
  prickling heat
  pustules, inflammed
Sneezing
Stupid, feeling
Teething

Thirst
  burning
  for cold drinks
Urine, muddy deposit

ACTR
Actea Racemosa
Black Cohosh

  Nervousness
  Restless, menses, during
  Sadness, menses, during

AESC
Aesculus Hippocastanum
Horse chestnut

  Backache
    lower down, severe
  Hemorrhoids
    blue grapes, like
    burning
  Hips, pain, aching, severe
  Rectum, dry

AGN-C
Agnus Castus
Chaste Tree

  Erections, absent
  Indifferent to everything
  Old looking
  Sadness
  Self-contempt

ALL-C
Allium Cepa
Onion

  Abdomen, pain, colicky
    from cucumbers
    from overeating
    from salad
    from wet feet
  Cough, as if tearing the larynx

Eyes, burning
  discharge, irritating
  running
  tearing
Hay fever, Fall worsens
  Spring worsens
Headache, air, open improves
  dull,evening worsens
Headache, dull,
  open air improves
  warm room worsens
Nose discharge,
  acrid
  bland
  burning
  irritating
  profuse
  watery
Sneezing, peaches, handling
    worsens
  rising worsens
Tears, irritating

ALOE
Aloe Socotrina
Socotrine Aloes

  Abdomen, pain,
    after stool improved
    before and during stool
    colicky
  Anus, burning,
      preventing sleep
    itching, preventing sleep
    pain, burning
      after drinking or
        eating
  Diarrhea
  Faintness after stool
  Flatus, burning
    offensive
  Hemorrhoids
    bleeding
    blue grapes, like

Hemorrhoids (cont'd.)
 hot
 itchy
 painful, cold water improves
Hemorrhoids, sore
 tender
Menses, early
Stool, urging to

ALUM
Alumina
Pure Clay

 Appetite for, chalk
  charcoal
  cloves
  coffee
  coffee grounds
  peculiar things
  starch
  tea grounds
 Chilliness
 Constipated
 Dryness
 Moon, full, worsens
  new worsens
 Periodicity, 14 days worsens
 Thin

AMBR-GR
Ambra Grisea
Ambergris

 Disinterested
  in everything
 Weeping, constant

ANT-C
Antimonion Crudum
Antimony Sulfide

 Appetite lost
 Face, eruption, red,
  patches, in new born
 Hair, rough

Measles, rash
Menses, early
Skin, rough scales
Thirst, excessive

APIS
Apis Mellifica
Honey Bee Poison

 Extremities, swelling of
 Eyes, swollen underneath
 Heat worsens
 Jealousy, complaints from
 Stings, bee
 Stuffy rooms worsen
 Swelling, warmth worsens
 Urination, frequent
  irritation on
 Urine, retention painful
  scalding

APOC
Apocynum Cannabinum
Indian Hemp

 Extremities, swollen after
  infection
 Thirsty
 Nausea, after drinking

APOM
Apomorphinum
An opium Alkaloid

 Nausea on motion

ARG-N
Argentum Nitricum
Silver Nitrate

 Anxiety in public places
 Appetite for sweets
 Chilliness
 Eyes, inflammation in
  new born

Faces, shriveled looking
Fear, going out in public
Gassy, after eating
Mind, tiredness of from
    overwork
Old looking
Restless
Thin
Throat, splinter sensation
    on swallowing
Diarrhea, from sugar
  in children
  like chopped spinach

ARIST
Aristolochia Clematitis
The Birthwort

Arthritis, menopausal
Childbirth eased
Epididymis inflamed
Gonorrhea
Happiness, alternates
    with sadness
Menses, before, worsened
  delayed
  prolonged
  short
Prostate inflamed
Sadness, alternates with
    happiness
Sexual desire
Skin conditions
Sterility
Stomach upsets
Urination, inflammation
Vagina, discharge
  discharge, brown
  discharge, slimy
  itching
Varicose veins

ARN
Arnica Montana

Leopard's Bane

Accident, unwell since an
Beaten, feels as if
Breasts, newborn, swollen
    after injury
Bruised feeling
Bruises
Childbirth, complaint of before
Ears, glands in front inflammed
Epilepsy, after injury
Erections, painful after injury
Eyes, inflammation, after injury
Face, eruption, red,
  patches in newborn
Falls
Injuries
Kidney disease from injury
Lameness
Operations, before
  effects of
Sitting, uncomfortable,
    because everything
    feels too hard
Skin, chafing in infants
Soreness
Sprains
Stiffness, from long riding
Stings wasp
Stool, foul
  frequent
  slimy
Tiredness
Vomiting blood
Weeping after coughing
Wounds, healing poor

ARS
Arsenicum Album
Arsenic Oxide

Abdomen, swollen
Anxiety
Appetite, for hot drinks
Asthma, cold drinks worsen

Asthma (cont'd.)
  leaning forward improves
  lying worsens
  midnight—2 a.m.
  walking improves
Breath, shortness, while lying
Burning pains
Chilliness, extreme
  Cold drinks worsen
  Cold drinks, worsens
    when overheated
Colic, from constipation
  from green food
Depressed
Despair
Diarrhea
  after cold drinks
    in hot weather
  after cold food in hot weather
  after drinking
  after eating
  night worse
  pain, burning
  painless
  2 a.m. worse
Eyes, blue circles around
Face, pale
  cheeks, sunburn
Fear, after midnight
  death
  disease is incurable
Hair falling
Hopeless, after midnight
Indifferent to everything
Influenza prevention
Intestinal colic from bad food
  colic from drinking cold water
Irritable
Legs, heels, discharges, frothy
  heels, eruption,
    bleeding on touch
  eruption, foul smelling
  eruption, grape-like
  eruptions, red, flat

Measles, itchy afterward
  rash, burning afterward
  rash, itching afterward
  rash, suppressed,
    vomiting follows
Menses, excessive
Midnight, after, worsens
Night, 2 a.m. worsens
Pains, burning like fire
Prostration
  profuse
Pulse frequent
  irregular
Restless
  after midnight
  extreme
Skin flabby
  hard patches
  loose
  scurfy patches
  ulcers with hard,
    red edges
Sleepless
Thirsty
Thirst for cold water
  in small sips
Tongue, red
Vagina, discharge, burning
  corrosive
  thin
Weak

ARS-I
Arsenicum Iodatum
Arsenic Iodide

Breathing, shortness of
Chilliness
Cough, hacking
Heart action, weak
  disease, organic
Open air improves
Weather, cold worsens
  dry worsens
  windy worsens

ARUM-T
Arum Triphyllum
Indian Turnip

Asthma
Lips, picking at
    upper, inflamed
Nose, discharge, acrid
    discharge, profuse
    inflamed
    inside, inflamed
    picking
Voice, hoarseness
    hoarse, singing worsens
    hoarse, talking worsens
    uncertain

AUR
Aurum Metallicum
Gold

Anxiety about the future
Appetite for coffee
Chilliness
Eyes, styes
Grief
Hopeless
Life, a burden
Memory poor
Palpitations, frequent
Suicidal
Tiredness

BACIL
Bacillinum
Tubercular Sputum

Cold preventative

BAPT
Baptisia Tinctoria
Wild Indigo

Expression, drunken
    stupid

Face, discoloration, dark
    red, dark
Limbs aching
Parts rested on feel sore
Prostration, profuse
Stupor
Throat, dark red
    putrid

BAR-C
Baryta Carbonica
Barium Carbonate

Depressed
Memory poor
Weakness, in children
    in old age

BELL
Belladonna
Deadly Nightshade

Chest, rattling in
Cough, barking
    dry
    hollow
    night worsens
Cuts
Eyes, sensitive to light
    watering
Fierceness, from sunstroke
Head, hot
    pulsation of
Headache
Limbs, jerking, sudden
Menses, between, worsens
    offensive
Mumps
Night, 2 a.m. worsens
Ovary, pain during menses
Pulse irregular
Respiration, difficult
    fast
Restless

Scarlet fever
Skin, dry
Sleepless
Sneezing, follows cough
Thirsty
Throat, rattling,
    during inspiration
Urination, frequency
    in pregnancy
Vagina, discharge, offensive
Voice, hoarseness
Vomiting
Weeping

BEL-P
Bellis Perennis
The Daisy

    Bruises
    Sprains
    Tiredness
    Wounds, deep
      infected

BLAT
Blatta Orientalis
Indian cockroach

    Extremities, swollen,
      after heart disease

BORX
Borax
Biborate of Soda

    Groin, pain
      pain during menses
    Menses, colicky
      early
      profuse
    Nausea
      on motion
      on descending

BROM
Bromium
Bromine

    Asthma, in blondes
      in sailors ashore

BRY
Bryonia Alba
Wild Hop

    Anger, worsens
    Appetite for hot drinks
    Backache, radiates
      along sciatic nerve
      cold bathing improves
    Breast, painful
      during pregnancy
    Brunettes
    Chest, pains, prickly
    Constipation, desire
      for stool absent
    Cough, dry
     frequent
     into gagging
     lying improves
     motion worsens
     warm room worsens
    Diarrhea, alternates
      with constipation
     warm weather causes
    Desires things immediately
     unobtainable things
    Dissatisfied with
      whatever offered
    Extremities stiff
    Gagging with cough
    Impatient
    Inhaling, grunting
    Intense people
    Irritable
    Joints, discoloration, redness
     hot
     pains, gouty

Joints (cont'd.)
  pains, motion worsens
  pains, stinging
  stiff
  swollen
  tender
Limbs, aching, motion worsens
Lips, cracked
  dry
Lying painful side improves
Measles, rash suppressed by
      cold, followed by
      respiration conditions
Motion, worsens
Mouth, dry
Painful parts, cold worsens
  lying on improves
Painful parts, perspiration
      improves
  touch worsens
Respiration, fast
  labored
Shoulder, discoloration, right
  pain, right radiating to
      upper arm
  swelling, right
Skin, prickling heat
Stomach, upsets from
      cold drinks and food
Stool, dark
  dry
  dry as if burnt
  large
Thirst, extreme
  large, in frequent amounts
  unquenchable
Tongue, cracked
  dry

BUFO
Bufo Rana
The Toad

Masturbation, excessive

CACT
Cactus Grandiflorus
Night-blooming Cereus

  Anger
  Breastbone, pain over
  Chest, constricting pain of
  Fear, of death
  Irritable
  Menses, painful, make her
      cry out
  Perspiration, cold
    profuse
  Pulse, weak

CADM
Cadmium Metallicum
Cadmium (the element)

  Influenza prevention

CALC
Calcarea Ostrearum
Oyster Shell

  Anxiety
  Breast, painful
  Breathing, shortness on
      exertion
  Cautious
  Chilliness
  Cold preventative
  Confused
  Convulsions, before measles
      eruption
  Depressed
  Despair
  Diaper rash, in chilly babies
  Eczema, wet
  Fatness
  Face, eruption, dry, with
      teething
  Fear of:
    being observed by others
    dark

Fear of (cont'd.)
  disaster
  disease
  insanity
Foot, pain
  cramping
  cramping, nighttime
Head, fontanelles swollen
  perspiration of
  night, soaking the pillow
Hopeless
Immobilized by fear
Joints, pains, climbing
        stairs worsens
  eating worsens
  motion worsens
  water worsens
Indifferent to everything
Legs, calves
  pain, cramping
  pain, nighttime
Limbs, cold, wet
Menses, early
  profuse
Night, 2 a.m. worsens
Perspiration, profuse
  after exertion, slight
Sadness
Skin, coldness, clammy
  discolored, pale
Speech, words misplaced
Sprain, cold worsens
  damp worsens
  exercise worsens
  warmth improves
Taste, sour with heartburn
Tiredness

CALC-F
Calcarea Fluorata
Flour Spar (calcium flouride)

  Childbirth eased
  Fingers, joints, swollen

Indigestion of pregnancy
Morning sickness in
        gassy persons
Wet pack improves
Wet weather worsens

CALC-P
Calcarea Phosphorica
Calcium Phosphate

  Bones, broken, healing of speeded
    non-uniting
  Erections, excessive
  Head, bones, brittleness of
        in children
    thinness of in children
    fontanelles, closing delayed
    fontanelles, reopen
        after closing
  Sexual desire excessive
  Teething, complicated
    delayed

CALEN
Calendula
Marigold

  Bleeding, after tooth
        extraction
    scalp wounds
  Childbirth, fear
  Exhaustion, from bleeding
    from pain
  Face, pale
  Inflammation, after injuries
  Joint fluid, lost by
        penetrating wounds
  Muscles ruptured
  Nerve tumors
  Tendons ruptured
  Wounds
    infections, prevention
    painful
  Wounds, infected
    ragged

CAMPH
Camphora
Camphor

Bed covers intolerable
Colds after chill
Pulse, weak
Skin, icy cold to touch

CAN-S
Cannabis Sativa
Hemp

Urination, painful
retarded
spurting

CANTH
Cantharides
Spanish Flies

Bladder, burning
on urination
Burns, blistered
Stings, infected
Urethra, burning
beginning of urination
close of urination
Urinary retention
Urination, burning
pain on
painful urgency
urging, painful after urination
Urine, bloody
retention painful
urgency constant

CAPS
Capsicum
Cayenne Pepper

Burns
Heartburn, of pregnancy

CARB-AN
Carbo Animalis
Animal Charcoal

Ankles turn on walking
Chilliness
Circulation poor
Hearing weak
Joints, sprained by slight
exertion
weak
Menses, flow only in a.m.
Muscles strained on
lifting smallest weight
Speech weak during menses
Weakness during the menses
general
of muscles

CARB-V
Carbo Vegetabilis
Vegetable Charcoal

Abdomen swollen with gas
belching improves
drinking worsens
eating worsens
lying down worsens
Air, fresh, desires
Appetite for salt
Belching, continuous
Chest pain
Cough, convulsive
evening worse
Exhausting diseases, effects of
Extremities, cold
Face, acne
Face, cold
pale
perspiring
pinched
Fanned, desires to be

Fanning improves
Fatty foods worsen
Fatigue
Flatus, loud
    smelly
Gassy
Memory poor
Perspiration, cold
Skin, blue
    eruption
Sleep, interrupted by
        cold extremities
Thinking slow
Weakness after anemia

CAUL
Caulophyllum
Blue Cohosh

Abdomen, pains during menses

CAUS
Causticum
Tinctura Acris Sine Kali

Angry before menses
Melancholy, before menses
Urination, leaking after
        coughing or sneezing

CEDR
Cedron
Simaba Cedron Seeds

Periodicity, daily time,
        same, worsens

CHAM
Chamomilla
Chamomile

Abdomen,swollen
Anger

Angry, beginning
    of menses
Anus, inflamed, during
    diarrhea
Appetite, for cold drink
Carried, babies improve
    only when
Colic, in infants, from anger
    from exposure to cold
Cough, day and night
    dry
    hoarse
Diaper rash, in restless, feverish babies
Diarrhea
Diarrhea, slimy, green
    smelly
Extremities, cold
Face, red
    swollen
Fretful, infants
    menses, during
Impressionable, menses, during
Irritable
Limbs, legs drawn against
        abdomen
    moving constantly
Measles, rash suppressed,
        vomiting follows
Menses, excessive, after anger
    excess after irritation
    painful
Peevish
Pelvis, pains, cramping
People, aversion to
Restless
Skin chafing in infants
    prickly heat
Spit
Stools, odor of rotten eggs
Teething, complicated
Weeping incessantly,
        holding improves

CHEL
Chelidonium Majus
Celandine

Hepatitis
Weakness after hepatitis

CINA
Cina
Worm Seed

Colic, in infants from worms
Nose, picking
Stool, worms

CINCH
Cinchona
Pevuvian Bark
Abdomen, rumbling
    swollen
Appetite for spices
Belching not improve
Chilliness, shivering from
Cough
Diarrhea, after drinking
    after eating
    night worsens
Flatus improves
Gassy
Gas from rectum
Headache
Influenza
Joints, pain
Legs, aching
Legs, swollen, watery,
        cold to touch
Menses, black clots
Nausea, at smell of food
    at thought of food
Periodicity
    7-14 days worsens
Perspiration, odor foul
    profuse
Salivation, profuse

Skin, yellow in newborn
Tiredness
Vomiting

COCC
Coccus Cacti
Cochineal Insect

Legs, weakness, before menses
Nausea, on sight of
        boat in motion
    riding in vehicle
Seasickness, menses during
Vertigo, menses during
Vomiting, on riding in a vehicle

COC-I
Cocculus
Cocculus Indicus

Appetite, lost
Constipation, from traveling
    from weariness
Head, back of, pain
    empty feeling, during
        seasickness
Mouth, taste metallic
Nausea, with dizziness
Speech difficult from weariness
Weariness, extreme

COFF
Coffea Cruda
Coffee

Calves, cramps during pregnancy
Chicken pox, anxiety after
    restlessness of
Teething

COLCH
Colchicum Automnale
Meadow Saffron

Anus, protrusion of

Colic, from green food
Gassy

COLOC
Colocynth
Squirting Cucumber

Abdomen, colicky pain
  after drinking
  after eating
  doubling up relieves
  stool relieves
Diarrhea, bloody
Extremities, restless
Stool, foul smelling
  sputtering
Thirsty

CON
Conium Maculatum
Poison Hemlock

Alone, aversion to being
Breasts, painful
  during pregnancy
Contradiction, cannot endure
Cough, night worsens
Disinterested, in business
  in everything
Domineering
Memory, poor
Menses, scanty
Quarrelsome
Sexual desire suppressed,
    complaints from
Society, avoids
Vertigo, lying down worsens
  turning in bed

CORR
Corallium Rubrum
Red Coral

Appetite, for sour

CROC
Crocus Sativus
Saffron

Menses, black shreds

CROT-CAS
Crotalus Cascavella
Brazilian Rattlesnake Venom

Clothing, averse to

CROT-H
Crotalus Horridus
Rattlesnake Venom

Bleeding, dark
Discoloration, bluish,
        of affected parts
  dusky, of affected parts
Dreams, of death
  of the dead
Face, discoloration, dark ·
Fingernails, discolored blue
Heart, turning over in chest,
    sensation
  weakness
Lying on right side worsens

CUPR
Cuprum Metallicum
Copper

Unconscious, from coughing
Vomiting after cough

CUPA
Cuprum Arsenicosum
Copper Arsenite

Calves, cramps during pregnancy
Respiration, wheezing during
  coughs

CYCL
Cyclamen Europaeum
Sow Bread

Headache
Menses, delayed in young girls
Open air worsens
Visual disturbances
Vertigo

DIG
Digitalis Purpurea
Foxglove

Chest, weakness on talking
Dying, feeling as if
Exhaustion
Eyelids, veins swollen
Faintness
Fingers, fall asleep
Heart, valves weak
Lips, veins swollen
Prostration, extreme
Pulse, slow
Skin, blue
    pale
Stomach, sinking in
Swelling, after Bright's
        disease
    after scarlet fever
Tongue, veins swollen
Urine, suppressed

DROS
Drosera Rotundifolia
Sundew

Cough, convulsive
    lying worsens
    motion improves
Vomiting after cough
Weak

DULC
Dulcamara
Bittersweet

Changing weather, worsens
Cold places worsen
Cold weather worsens
Cough, after cold exposure
    after damp exposure
Dampness worsens
Ear, glands below inflamed
    glands in front inflamed
    inflamed
Hayfever, from cold
    from wading in cold water
    from weather changing
        hot to cold
    from wet weather
Kidney disease from
        exposure to dampness
Rheumatism, acute
Spit, expelled easily
Wet weather worsens

EUCAL
Eucalyptus
Blue Gum (Fever tree)

Aching
Asthma
Colds
Cough, influenzal
Influenza
Nose, discharge, foul
    discharge, irritating
Stiffness
Tiredness

EUP
Eupatorium Perfoliatum
Boneset

Bones, aching
    broken feeling

Bones (cont'd.)
  bruised feeling
Eyeballs sore
Influenza
Nose, running

EUPHR
Euphrasia
Eyebright

Bed worsens
Cough, daytime
  moist
  night worsens
  south wind worsens
  tobacco smoke worsens
  with gagging
Eyes, discharge, bland
  inflammation
  tearing, morning on rising
Gagging with cough
Indoors worsens
Nose, discharge, irritating
  discharge, morning on rising
Warmth, worsens

FERR
Ferrum Metallicum
Iron

Appetite for bread
Calves, cramps during pregnancy
Menses, increased
Vomiting after coughing
  after meals

FER-P
Ferrum Phosphoricum
Ferric Phosphate

Cold improves
Joints, pain
  pains, motion worsens
Motion, worsens

Swelling, red

FICS
Ficus Religiosa
Pakur (from India)

Menses, bright red
  profuse

FLAC
Fluoric Acid
Hydrofluoric Acid

Appetite for spices

FORM-R
Formica Rufa
The Ant

Stings, ants

GELS
Gelsemium
Yellow Jasmine

Backache
Back, bruised feeling
Chilliness
Confused
Coordination, muscular, lack of
Dampness, worsen
Depressed
Desires, to be left alone
Dizziness
Emotional excitement,
  complaints from
Headache, band-like around
  the head
  during menses
  painful in young girls
Muscles, not obey will
Pains, aching
Staggering, on motion of the head
Tired, so speech impossible

Trembling, from weakness
Walking, with difficulty
Weak

GLON
Glonine
Nitroglycerine

Face, red
Head, swollen, feeling
Headache, from sunrise to sunset
    heat worsens
    jarring worsens
    pulsating
    pulsation of blood worsens
    stepping worsens
    throbbing
Stroke, from heat
Sun worsens

GRAPH
Graphites
Black Lead

Constipated
Face, acne
Genital itching before menses
Menopause

HAM
Hamamelis Virginica
Witch Hazel

Bleeding, bad effects of
Bruises
Burns, blistered
Eyes, inflammation of
            conjunctiva
Injuries from falls
Menses, dark
Ovaries, painful
Wounds, bruised
    ragged (torn)

HEP
Hepar Sulphur
Sulphuret of Lime

Anger
Anxiety
Appetite, for sour
        for spices
Breasts, newborn, swollen,
            after injury
Burns, infected
Chest, rattling in with cough
Chilliness
Cold, sensitive to
Complaining
Cough, choking
    croupy
    daytime
    dry
Cough, west wind worsens
Diaper rash in chilly babies
Drafts worsen
Face, acne
Hypochondriasis
Injuries, infected
Irritable
Mange
Sensitivity, extreme
Sensitive to light
Touch, sensitive to
Weeping, after coughing

HYOS
Hyoscyamos Niger
Henbane

Excitable
Jealousy, complaints from
Urinary retention
Urination, pain on
    painful urging
    retention painful

HYPER
Hypericum Perforatum
St.John's Wort

Back, injury to
Changing weather worsens
Coccyx, pain from falls on
Cold, worsens
Concussion, from injury
Dampness worsens
Depression, after fright
  after operation
Emotional, after injuries
  or operation
Erections, poor after
  spinal injury
Fear, complaints from
Fog, worsens
Headaches, from spinal injury
Hypnotism, complaints from
Injuries, crushing
Jarring, sensitive to
Menses, difficult from injuries
  to coccyx
Motion, sensitive to
Nerve injuries
Ovaries, illness following
  injuries to coccyx
Shock, complaints from
Spine, injuries to
Touch, of injured part, sensitive to
Weakness, from worry
Wounds, from sharp instrument

IGN
Ignatia
St. Ignatius Bean

Constipated
Despair
Grief
Hopeless
Nervousness

Numbness
Oversensitive to pain
Sighing involuntarily
Throat, ball sensation of
Tobacco smoke worsens

IOD
Iodum
Iodine

Air, fresh, desires
Appetite, insatiable
  ravenous
Asthma, cold air improves
  in brunettes
  warmth worsens
Breathing shortness, on exertion
Constipated
Heart palpitations, squeezed
  rapidly, as if
Heat worsens
Thin
Warmth, in women, worsens
Weak
Weakness, profound
Weight, loss (thin)

IP
Ipecacuanha
Ipecac

Asthma
Bleeding, bright red
Breathing, labored
Chest, tightness of
Colic in infants, from
  fatty foods
Cough, dry
  fatiguing
  paroxysms
  whooping
Diarrhea, blood-streaked
  cold weather causes

Diarrhea (cont'd.)
  strange food causes
  with vomiting
Face pale
Gagging, with asthma
Measles, rash suppressed,
      vomiting follows
Menses, bright red
Mouth, salivation
Nausea constant
Restless
Stomach, vomiting with cough
Stools, putrid
Vagina, discharge, bright red
      between menses
Vomiting
  mucous, shiny white
  with asthma
  with diarrhea

KALI-BI
Kali Bichromicum
Potassium Bichromate

Burns, ulcerated
Cough, croupy
  in chilly children
Face, acne
Gastric complaints from
      cold drinks on hot days
Heat worsens
Mucous, stringy
  tough
  viscid
Nose, discharge plugs
Sinus trouble

KALI-C
Kali Carbonicum
Potassium Carbonate

Eyelids, upper, swollen
Loins, dragging
  weakness

KALI-S
Kali Sulfuricum
Potassium Sulfate

Air, fresh, improves
Evening worsens
Heat worsens
Joint pains, heat worsens
  shifting from place to place
  swollen
Tongue, yellow-coated

KREO
Kreosotum
Kreosote

Irritable, before menses
Restless, before menses

LACH
Lachesis
Surukuku Snake Venom

Appetite, for salt
Clothing, averse to
Diarrhea, alternates with
      constipation
  black
  sticky
  white
Heat worsens
Menopause
Morning, worse in
Pressure
Sided, left, worsens
Skin, sensitive to least touch
Sleep, after worsened
Touch, worsens

LAT-M
Latrodectus Mactans
Black Widow Spider

Fear, dying by inability
  to breathe

Gasping in pain
Heart, pain, extending to left
    extending to left arm
    extending to shoulders
    severe
Pulse, frequent
    weak

LED
Ledum Palustre
Marsh Tea

Ankles, weak
Bites, animal
Chilliness
Eyes, bruising injuries to
    discoloration from injury
Injured areas feel cold
    to the touch
Jarring, sensitive to
Motion, sensitive to
Nerve injuries
Pains, cold improves
Poisonous bites
Skin, black and blue bruises
Sprains
Stings, insect
Warmth, worsens
Wounds from sharp instrument

LIL-T
Lilium Tigrinum
Tiger Lily

Busyness, from sexual repression
Cursing
Depressed
Despair
Fear
Hopeless
Hurried but without point
Listless
Moods alternate
Obscene speech

Restless
Sided, left, worsens
Striking at others
Timid
Walking, aversion to
Weeping

LYC
Lycopodium Clavatum
Club Moss

Abdomen, rumbling
    rumbling, audible
        across the room
    swollen, painful
Afternoon, worse at 4 p.m.
Air, fresh desires
Alone, aversion to being
Anger
Angry, before menses
Ankles, swollen, from
        heart disease
Appetite, for sweets
    increased after meals
Argumentative
Back, small of, pain as if breaking
Belching
    after meals
    worse at 4 p.m.
Bossy
Contradiction, cannot endure
    worsens
Critical of others
Erèctions, poor
Extremities, numbness
Face, eruptions, oozing
        with teething
Fear, being alone
Flatus, loud
    smelly
Food tastes sour
Gassy
    after eating

Hands, numbness
Headache, from hunger
Intellectuals
Irritable
Joint pains, heat worsens
   motion improves
   sided, right
   rest worsens
Melancholy before menses
Opposition, cannot endure
Peevish
Public appearances, worse before
Sided, right, worsens
Skin chafing in infants
Tests, worse before
Weakness, in old age
   in children
   physical
Worrisome

MAG-C
Magnesia Carbonica
Magnesium Carbonate

Backache before menses
Belching, sour
Chilliness
Menses, black
   delayed
   night worsens
   tarry
Odor, sour
Pains, bearing down,
         before menses
Sour disposition
Uterus, dragging pain
   dragging pain extending
      to genitals
Weakness before menses

MAG-M
Magnesia Muriatica
Magnesium Chloride

Irritable before menses

MAG-P
Magnesia Phosphorica
Magnesium phosphate

Menses, painful, hot
      applications relieve
   painful in attacks

MED
Medorrhinum
Gonorrheal Tissue

Daytime worsens
Foot, ball of painful/soreness
Heat worsens
Joint pains, shifting
      from place to place
Joints, cracking
   stiff on walking
Motion worsens
Night improves
Seashore improves
Shoulders, pain
   pain, left side
Sun worsens
Thunderstorms worser

MERC
Mercurius
Mercury

Anus, protrusion after stool
   redness
Appetite, for cold drink
   for dirt
   for foul things
   for horse dung
Breath, offensive
Chicken pox, after fever
      has passed
Chilliness, shivering from
Colic, in infants
Cough, dry
   violent

Diarrhea, cold weather causes
  with teething
Face, eruptions, discharging,
  irritating
Fever, alternating with chills
Gums, sore
Hair, falling
Influenza, horses
Legs, heels, eruptions,
  ulcers
Mouth, ulcers
Mumps
Neck, glands, swollen
Nose discharge, profuse
  discharge watery
  soreness
Perspiration, excessive
  night
  profuse
  profuse, night
Salivation, profuse
Scarlet fever
Shivering
Skin chafing, in infants
  leaden color in baldspots
  yellow in newborn
Stools, sour odor
  watery
Urination, profuse
Voice, hoarseness with cough

MORB
Morbillinum
Measles Tissue

Measles, complications of

MUR-AC
Muriatic Acid
Hydrochloric Acid

Hemorrhoids, protrude
    during urination
    tender on least touch

NAJA
Naja Naja Naja
Cobra Venom

Brooding, over imaginary
  troubles
Death, desires own
Heart, action excited
  enlarged
  heaving
  pain, cramping
  cramping, extending to
    left neck
  cramping, extending to
    left shoulder
  cramping extending to
    left shoulder blade
  lying on left side worsens
  open air improves
  pain, stitching
  weakness from previous disease
  weakness in, feeling of
Lying left side worsens
Pulse, irregular intensity

NAT-M
Natrum Muriaticum
Common Salt

Appetite, for bread
  for salt
Back, small of, bruised feeling
  small of, lame feeling
Cold preventative
Constipated
Face, earthy complexion
Faintness, before menses
Hair falling
Hayfever, from heat
  from sun
Heat worsens
Homosexuality, female
Irritable
Joints, cracking
  pain, tearing on standing

Joints (cont'd.)
    pain, tearing on walking
Joints, pains, stinging
    on standing
    stinging on walking
Mange
Menses, scanty
Nose, as if worm crawling inside
Scrawny (thin)
Seashore worsens
Spit, bloody
Sun worsens
Taste, sour
Thin
Toe, discolored red
    swollen
Warmth, feeling of
Weeping, causeless

NATS
Natrum Sulphuricum
Sodium Sulfate

Appetite, for cold drinks

NIT-AC
Nitric Acid
Nitric Acid

Backache
Hemorrhoids,
    bleed on touch
    painful after stool
    like needles
Pelvis, pains, bearing down
Restless, midnight, after
Thighs, pain in
Urine, smell like horses' urine
Vagina, bleeding at menopause
    miscarriage, after

NUX-M
Nux Moschata
Nutmeg

Absent-minded

Appetite for coffee
Fatigue
Indifferent to everything
Memory, poor for
    familiar things
Moods swing widely
Sensitive, to light
    noise
    odors
    touch
Sleepiness, overpowering
Speech, wrong words in
Thinking, poor
Thoughts, vanish while reading
    while talking
    while writing
Weakness, in old age

NUX-V
Nux Vomica
Poison Nut

Abdomen, hernia, in newborn
Anger
Anus, protrusion after stool
Appetite, for spices
Belching
Brunettes
Calves, cramps during pregnancy
Chilliness
Coffee worsens
Colic, from constipation
    in infants
Constipated
Constipation alternating
    with diarrhea
Cough, dry
Cough, fatiguing
    paroxysms
Diarrhea, alternates with
    constipation
    cold weather cause
    slimy
Flanks bloated

Flatus, loud
  painful
Fretful
Gassy
Gas after eating
Hemorrhoids
  cold bathing improves
  constipation, from
  itchy
Intellectuals
Intense people
Irritable
Morning, worse in
Morning sickness
Motion worsens
Nausea, after eating
  morning
  vomiting relieves
Quarrelsome
Scarlet fever
Sensitive, to alcohol
  coffee
  criticism
  everything
  light
  mental exertion
  music
  noise
  odors
  people
  spices
  tobacco smoke
  touch
Sleepiness, early in evening
Stomach, heavy feeling
  upsets from coffee, tobacco,
    alcohol, or spicy foods
  vomiting with cough
Taste, bitter
  sour
Thin
Tobacco smoke worsens
Tongue, brown-coated
  coated white

Tongue (cont'd.)
  coated yellow
  tip, red
Urination, frequency in pregnancy
Vomiting, during cough
  food as soon as it hits stomach
Waking, 3-4 a.m.

OP
Opium
Poppy

Constipation, desire for
    stool absent
Delirious
Epilepsy, as if dead after
Eyes half-closed
Immobile
Limbs, moving constantly
Perspiration, profuse and hot
Respiration, labored
  stertorous
Stool, dark
  dry
  hard

ORIG
Origanum Marjorana
Sweet Marjoram

Masturbation, excessive
Sexual desire, excessive
  in women

PARTID
Parotidinium
Mumps Bacteria

Mumps, complications

PERTUS
Pertussin
Whooping Cough Bacteria

Cough, whooping, bad effects

PETR
Petroleum
Coal Oil

Nausea, of pregnancy
   continuous

PHOS
Phosphorus
Phosphorus

Appetite, for cold drinks
   for cold food
   for salt
Burning pains
Cough, chronic
   cold air worsens
   drinking worsens
   eating worsens
   laughing worsens
   lying on left side worsens
   reading worsens
   talking worsens
Depressed before menses
Diarrhea
Eyes, blue circles around
Expression, hangdog
Face, pale
   wizened
Fear, thunder
Fidgety
Gloomy, about future
Homosexuality, male
Indifferent to everything
Masturbation, excessive
Measles, rash suppressed,
      chest affected
Sensitive, to everything
   lights
   noise
   odors
   touch
Sexual desire excessive
Speech, slowly answers
Stupor

Throat, windpipe painful
Thunderstorms worsen
Tiredness
Ulcers, bleeding
Voice, hoarseness
Weak
Weary of life
Withdrawn from life

PHOS-AC
Phosphoric Acid
Glacial Phosphoric Acid

Chagrin, complaints from
Disinterested in everything
Erections absent after
      sexual excesses
Grief from unhappy
      love affair
Homesickness
Listless
Indifferent to everything
Thinking slow
Tiredness
Weakness, from grief
   in old age
Weeping
Withdrawn from life

PIC-AC
Picric Acid
Picric Acid

Activity, emotional or
      mental worsens
Erections, long-lasting
   violent
Masturbation, excessive
Sexual desire, excessive
Tiredness

PLAT
Platinum
Platinum

Gay and sad alternately

Genitalia hypersensitive
  to touch
Haughty
Intercourse painful
Menses, clotted, dark
  early
  profuse
Pride, worsens
Sexual desire excessive
    in women

PLUM
Plumbum
Lead

Appetite for bread
Vagina, constriction of

PODO
Podophyllum
May Apple

Diarrhea, bathing, during
  chronic
  early a.m. to noon
  early morning
  eating, after
  in teething children
  painless
Stool, foul-smelling
  green
  profuse
  watery

PSOR
Psorinum
A Scabies Vesicle

Asthma, lying flat improves
Body odor
Chilliness, extreme
Delusion of being
    fatally ill
Despair
Diarrhea, foul-smelling
    like decayed flesh

Drafts, cold, worsens
Face, sickly
Fear, of business failure
  death
  disease is incurable
  everything
  future
  religious salvation
Hay fever
  previous history of asthma
    or eczema
  returns yearly at same day
Hopeless
Mange
Sadness
Suicidal

PULEX
Pulex Irritans
Flea

Bites, flea

PULS
Pulsatilla
Anemone

Action slow
Air, fresh, desires
  fresh, improves
Affectionate
Blondes
Changing symptoms
Closed rooms worsen
Colic, in infants, from
    fatty foods
  infants with gas
  infants with vomiting
Cough, loose
Desires fresh air
Diarrhea, night worsens
Ear inflamed
Eyes, running
  styes
Fatty foods worsen

Fickle
Food, fatty, worsens
Fresh air improves
Gentle
Heartburn, of pregnancy
Hives
Laughing easily
Measles, rash suppressed,
    diarrhea follows
Menses, black
  clotted
  delayed in young girls
  intermittent, in young girls
  scanty
  suppressed from wet feet
Mild disposition
Miscarriage, threatened
Morning sickness after fats
  fresh air improves
Mouth, dry
Nausea
Nose, discharge, colored
  discharge thick
Obese
Open air improves
Pains, shifting
Scarlet fever
Skin, burning in spots
  discoloration, red spots
  dry
  eruptions
  eruptions, cool bathing
      improves
  eruptions, from eating fats
  eruptions, for eating pork
  hot
  prickling
Sneezing
Stuffy rooms worsen
Taste, foul
Testicles inflamed in mumps
Thinking, slow
Thirsty
Thirstless
Timid

Tongue moist and white
Urination, frequency
  in pregnancy
Urine, scanty
Voice, hoarseness
Vomiting, after cough
Warmth worsens
Weeping
Wind worsens
Women, diseases of

RHOD
Rhododendron
Snowrose

  Changing weather worsens
  Fear, thunder
  Stormy weather worsens
  Storm, before, worsens
  Wind worsens

RHUS-T
Rhus Toxicodendron
Poison Ivy

  Alcohol worsens
  Abdomen, perspiration of
  Arthritis, wet weather worsens
    winter worsens
  Backache, radiates along
        sciatic nerve
    radiates to leg
  Back, small of, aching
    stiffness, as if from a blow
    stiff, as if sprained
  Bed feels too hard
  Chest, heaving of
  Cold worsens
  Eyes, inflammation, cold worsens
    damp worsens
    in newborn, on waking,
        improved by activity
  Extremities, alternately
        hot and cold
    numbness, where lain upon
  Face, eruption, crusty at teething

Joints, pains, cold weather
 worsens
 drafts worsen
 heat improves
 massage, gentle, improves
 motion improves
 motion, continued, improves
 pains, motion, first, on
 pains, night time
 pains, wet weather worsens
 stiff, morning, on rising
Leg, swollen, watery, hot to touch
 watery, stiff
Measles, skin tender after
Motion, first worsens but better
 by continued motion
Nose, inflamed
 pain on touch
 red
Poison ivy protection
Restless
Restlessness, physical
Shoulders, pain
 stiff, as if sprained
Skin, inflammation
 patches, hard
 patches, raised
 ring worm
 scabby
 scabs reform if removed
Sprains, cold worsens
 damp worsens
 exercise improves
 rest worsens
 warmth improves
Swelling, red
 shiny
 smooth
Urination, frequent

RHUS-V
Rhus Venenata
Poison Sumack

 Foot, ball of, pain, shooting

Foot (cont'd.)
 bones of, pain, shooting
 heel, pains

RUTA
Ruta Graveolens
Rue

 Bones, broken, bruised
  crushed
  bruised
  pain, deep
 Bruised feeling
 Changing position
  constantly from pain
 Dislocations
 Parts rested on feel sore
 Sprains
  cold worsens
  damp worsens
  exercise improves
 Sprains, pain of, extending
  to bones
  rest worsens
  warmth improves

SABAD
Sabadilla
Ceyadilla

 Eyes, watering
 Eyelids, burning
  discolored, red
 Face, hot
 Nose, discharge
 Skin, dry
 Sneezing, paroxysms
 Throat, dry

SABN
Sabina
Savine

 Menses, bright red
  paroxysms
  standing improves
  walking improves

SANG
Sanguinaria
Blood Root

    Appetite for spices
    Breasts, painful, stitching
    Nipples, burning
      sore

SEC
Secale Cornutum
Ergot

    Legs, heels, discharges, frothy
      eruption, bleeding on touch
      foul smelling
      grape-like
      red, flat
    Menses, dark
      fluid

SENC
Senecio Aureus
Squaw-Weed (Golden Ragwort)

    Menses, irregular
      painful
      scanty

SEP
Sepia Officinalis
Cuttle Fish

    Appetite for sour
    Childbirth, complaints after
    Chilliness, after cold wind
    Colds, frequent
      worsen
    Constipated
    Depressed
    Ears, pain in cold wind
    Eczema, creases of extremities
      dry
    Eczema, itching
      summer improves
      winter worsens

Evening worsens
Extremities cold
Face, acne
    eruption, red, patches in
      new born
    sallow
Fingers, skin cracked in winter
Hair, dull
    falling
    stringy
Heat, flushes at
    flashes, monopausal
Indifferent to loved ones
Indolence
Intercourse, painful
Irritable, before menses
Joints, cracking
    pains, heat improves
    menopausal
    sided, left
    stiff
    weakness of, profound
Lesbianism
Mange
Menopause
Menses, before, worse
    clotted
    frequent
    infrequent
    irregular
    long
    profuse
    prolonged
    scanty
    short
    thin
    worsened before
Miscarriage
    first three months
    threatened
Nausea, at smell of food
    at thought of food
    motion of cars
    of pregnancy, from motion

Nausea (cont'd.)
  of pregnancy, morning
Nose, discoloration, greenish-yellow
    over bridge
Pains, bearing down, before menses
Pelvic organs, as if falling out
  heat of ascending
Sadness
Sallowness
Sexual desire lost
Sided, left, worsens
Skin, blisters watery
  blisters, whitish
  discolored, sallow
  odor, fishy
  oily
  ringworm
  tender when touched
Sterility
Tiredness
Urination, night in bed
Vagina, pains on intercourse
Weakness after anemia
Weeping, menses, before
Wind, cold worsens
  worsens

SIL
Silicea
Quartz

  Appetite, for cold drink
  Chilliness
  Colds after chilled feet
  Cold worsens
  Emotionally passive
  Fear, before exams
  Fears everything
  Feet, chilliness, icy
  Head, fontanelles swollen
  Indigestion
  Infections heal slowly
  Introversion
  Nails, malformed, twisted

Not finish projects
Quitters
Shy
Skin infected easily
Stubborn
Tiredness, from slight exertion
Unsure of self
Urination, night in bed
Weakness, in children
  muscles

SPIG
Spigelia
Pinkroot

  Heart, pain, cold weather
    worsens
  compressing
  motion worsens
  severe
  sticking
  wet weather worsens
  palpitations, audible
  palpitations, violent
  Pulse, irregular
  Sensitive to touch

SPONG
Spongia Tosta
Roasted Sponge

  Anxiety
  Asthma, inspiration worsens
    with cough
  Cough, cold drinks worsen
    drafts worsen
    lying worsens
    wind worsens
    with asthma
  Faintness
  Heart pain
    pain, constricting
    palpitations
  Perspiration

Respiration gasping after
    midnight
suffocating sensation

STAN
Stannum
Tin

Chest, empty sensation
    weak sensation
Cough, evening in bed
    laughing worsens
    paroxysms of three
    singing worsens
    talking worsens
    warm drinks worsen
Sadness
Spit, greenish-yellow
    profuse
    salty
    sweet
Weeping

STAPH
Staphisagria
Stavesacre

Anger
    repressed, complaints from
        worsens
Bites, mosquito
Bladder inflamed, in brides
Chagrin, complaints from
Cold drinks worsen
Dissatisfied with whatever offered
Eyes, styes
Envy worsens
Grief
Hostile, suppressed, worsens
Indignation
Injuries, from sharp instruments
Intercourse, painful
Morning, worse in
Mortification, complaints from

Pain, cutting
    smarting
    stinging
Pride, worsens
Rage, suppressed, worsens
Sensitive, to emotional hurt
Sleepless all night, sleepy in
    daytime
Touch, of injured part, sensitive to
Vagina, painful, from pressure
    of clothes
Warmth improves
Wounds, from sharp instruments

STROP
Strophanthus Hispidus
Onáye (Irée)

Breathing, shortness of
Fingers, heaviness
Forearms, heaviness of
Heart action excited
Heart failure
Nausea
Pulse, frequent
    irregular rate
    weak
Secretions increased
Stomach, burning
Throat, burning
Vomiting
Twitching, of body

SUL
Sulfur
The Element, Sulfur

Air, fresh, desires
Anus, redness
    soreness
Appetite, for cold drinks
    spices
    sweets
Bathing, averse to

Chest, rattling in
  expectoration improves
Constipated, from painful stool
  with unsuccessful desire for stool
Cough, dry
Desires fresh air
Diarrhea, chronic
  morning, early
  painless
  protracted
  with teething
Diaper rash, in hot babies
Dirty
Eyes, inflammation
  inflammation in new born
  styes
Face, eruption, eyebrows,
    with teething
  red
Faintness, before lunch
Flatus, smelling like rotten eggs
Heat, flushes
Head, fontanelles swollen
  hot
Heat flashes, in evening
  worsens
Heated, feels
Hemorrhoids
  bathing worsens
  burning
  cold air improves
  itching
  scratching worsens
  recurrent
  standing worsens
Hot, feels
Influenza
Irritable
Leg, eruption, itchy
  oozing
  scurfy
Mange
Measles, burning afterward
  fever

Measles (cont'd.)
  itchy afterward
  rash, burning afterward
  itchy afterwards
Menses, absent
  delayed
  scanty
Restless, physical
Scarlet fever
Skin, chafing in infants
  eruptions
  odor of rotten eggs
Skin, prickling heat
  ringworm
Sleepiness, early in evening
Spit, green
  lumpy
Standing worsens
Stool, dry
  foul
  hard, as if burnt
  knotty
  large
  painful
Stuffy rooms worsen
Sun worsens
Thirst for cold drinks
Uncovers feet at night
Warmth, worsens
Weakness, after hepatities

SUL-AC
Sulfurous Acid
Sulfurous Acid

  Pollution, air

SYMPH
Symphytum
Comfrey

  Bones, broken
    pain, prickling
    pain from old injuries
    shaft, pain along

Eyeballs, pain from bruise
Nausea of pregnancy with
    retching

TAB
Tabacum
Tobacco

Air, fresh, improves
Chilliness with cold perspiration
Despondent
Diarrhea
Dizzyness, on closing the eyes
Headache, early morning
Heart, pain, twisting
    palpitations
Nausea, air, cold, improves
    fresh, improves
    motion worsens
    of pregnancy, continuous
Perspiration, cold
    with chilliness
Stomach, faint feeling in
    sinking in
Sweat, cold
Vomiting
    air, fresh, improves
    motion worsens
Weak

TARANT
Tarantula
Tarantula

Stings, spider

TART
Tartaricum Acidum
Tartaric Acid

Chest, rattling in
Diarrhea with cough
Vomiting, night
Weakness, with cough

THALAS
Thalaspi Bursa Pastoris
Shepherd's Purse

Menses, clotted
    hemorrhage, like a
Tiredness

THUJ
Thuja Occidentalis
White Cedar

Extremities, cracking when
    stretched
    stretching frequently
Leg, eruptions, itching
    oozing
    scruffy
    heels, discharges, frothy
    heels, eruptions, bleeding
        on touch
    foul smelling
    grape-like
    red, flat
Skin, hard patches
    pimples

TUB
Tuberculinum
Tubercle Bacillus

Changing weather worsens
Colds, frequent
    from open air
Ears, oozing behind
Eczema, itching while
        undressing
    white
    bran-like
    itching at night
Face, acne
    pale
Milk worsens
Scalp, oozing of

Skin folds, ooze
   troubles
Weakness with tubercular
   family history

URT-U
Urtica Urens
Stinging Nettle

Burns, simple
Ears, swollen shut
Eyes, swollen
Lips, swollen shut
Nose, swollen shut
Skin, eruptions, itching
   hot
   numbness
   tingling
Stings, bee
Urine, dark
   profuse
   uric acid crystals

USTL
Ustilago Maidis
Corn-Smut

Menses, excessive
Vagina, bleeding after menses
   bleeding before menses

VALE
Valeriana
Valerian

Depressed
Irritable
Sleepless

VARIC
Varicella
Chicken Pox Virus

Chicken Pox, complications

VERAT-A
Veratrum Album
White Hellebone

Abdomen, cold feeling in
Appetite for sours
Chilliness, extreme
Cholera
Collapse
Diarrhea, before menses
   profuse with vomiting
Disinterested in everything
Ears, coldness
Extremities, coldness to touch
Fainting, at least exertion
Forehead, cold perspiration of
Motion, slow
Nausea before menses
Nervousness
Plunges downwards
Prostration, profound
Pulse, rapid
Skin, cold to touch
   icy cold to touch
Staggering
Thirst for ice cold water
Trembling
Urination, involuntary with cough
Vomiting, with profuse diarrhea
Weakness, after the menses
   during the menses
   whole body

VESP
Vespa Vulgaris
The Wasp

Stings, wasp

VIBUR
Viburnum Opulus
High Cranberry Bush

Menses, cramping pain

Pelvis, pains, cramping

VIOL
Viola Odorata
The Violet

Face, eruption, pustules at
    teething
Urine, smell offensive

XANT
Xanthoxylum
Prickly Ash

Delicate women
Menses, early
  painful
  profuse

X-RAY
X-Ray
X-ray

Burns, x-ray

SECTION III
SYMPTOM GUIDE

SYMPTOM GUIDE

Abdomen, cold feeling in VERAT-A
  hernia in new born NUX-V
  pain after drinking or eating
    ALOE, COLOC
    stool improved ALOE
   before and during stool ALOE
  colicky ALL-C, ALOE, COLOC
    from cucumber ALL-C
    from overeating ALL-C
    from salad ALL-C
    from wet feet ALL-C
   doubling up relieves COLOC
   during menses CAUL
  perspiration of RHUS-T
  rumbling CINCH, LYC
   audible across the room LYC
  swollen ARS, CHAM, CINCH
Abdomen, swollen, painful LYC
  with gas CARB-V
Absent-minded NUX-M
Accident, unwell since an ARN
Aching EUCAL
Action, slow PULS
Activity, emotional or mental
    worsens PIC-AC
Affectionate PULS
Afternoon, 4 p.m. worse at LYC
Air, fresh, desires CARB-V, IOD,
  LYC, PULS, SUL

Air, fresh (cont'd.)
  improves ACON, KALI-S,
    PULS, TAB
Alcohol worsens RHUS-T
Alone, aversion to being CON, LYC
Anger BRY, CACT, CHAM, HEP,
  LYC, NUX-V, STAPH
  before menses CAPS, LYC
Anger, beginning of menses CHAM
  repressed, complaints from STAPH
  worsens BRY, STAPH
Ankles, swollen from heart disease LYC
Ankles, turn on walking CARB-AN
  weak LED
Anus, burning, preventing sleep ALOE
  inflamed during diarrhea CHAM
  itching, preventing sleep ALOE
  pain, burning ALOE
  protrusion of COLCH
   after stool MERC, NUX-V
  redness MERC, SUL
  soreness SUL
Anxiety: ACON, ARS, CALC,
  HEP, SPONG
  about the future AUR
  in public places ARG-N
Appetite
  for:
    bread FERR, NAT-M, PLUMB

Appetite (cont'd.)
  for: (cont'd.)
    chalk, ALUM
    charcoal ALUM
    Cloves ALUM
    coffee ALUM, AUR, NUX-M
    coffee grounds ALUM
    cold drinks, CHAM, MERC,
                NAT-S, PHOS, SIL, SUL
    cold foods PHOS
    dirt MERC
    foul things MERC
    horse dung MERC
    hot drinks ARS, BRY
    peculiar things ALUM
    salt CARB-V, LAC-C, NAT-M,
                PHOS
    sours, SEP
    spices CINCH, FL-AC,
                HEP, NUX-V, SANG, SUL
    starch ALUM
    sweets ARG-N, LYC, SUL
    tea grounds ALUM
  increased after meals LYC
  insatiable IOD
  lost ACON, ANT-C, COC-1
  ravenous IOD
Argumentative LYC
Arthritis, menopausal ARIST
  wet weather worsens RHUS-T
  winter worsens RHUS-T
Asthma ARUM-T, EUCAL, IP
  cold air improves IOD
  drinks worsen ARS
  in blondes BROM
    brunettes IOD
    sailors ashore BROM
  inspiration worsens SPONG
  leaning foward improves ARS
  lying flat improves PSOP
    worsens ARS
  midnight to 2 a.m. ARS
  walking improves ARS
  warmth worsens IOD

Backache AESC, GELS, NIT-AC,
                RHUS-T
  as if from a blow RHUS-T
  before menses MAG-C
  low down, severe AESC
  radiates along sciatic nerve RHUS-T
    cold bathing improves BRY
  to leg RHUS-T
Back, bruised feeling GELS
  injuries to HYPER
  small of, aching RHUS-T
    bruised feeling NAT-M
    lame feeling NAT-M
    pain, as if breaking LYC
    stiff, as if from a blow RHUS-T
    as if sprained RHUS-T
Bathing, averse to SUL
Beaten, feels as if ARN
Bed covers intolerable CAMPH
  feels too hard RHUS-T
Bed worsens EUPHR
Belching CARB-V, LYC, NUX-V
  after meals LYC
  continuous CARB-V
  not improve CINCH
  sour MAG-C
  worse 4 p.m. LYC
Bites, animal LED
  flea PULEX
  mosquito STAPH
Bladder burning CANTH
  on urination CANTH
  inflammation in brides STAPH
Bleeding, after tooth extractions CALEN
  bad effects of HAM
  bright red IP
  dark CROT-H
  scalp wounds CALEN
Blondes PULS
Body odor PSOR
Bones, aching EUP
  broken SYMPH
    bruised RUTA

Bones (cont'd.)
  broken (cont'd.)
    crushed RUTA
    feeling EUP
    healing of, speeded CALC-P
    nonuniting CALC-P
    pain, pricking SYMPH
  bruised feeling EUP
  bruises RUTA
  pain, deep RUTA
Bone pain from old injuries SYMPH
  shaft, pain along SYMPH
Bossy LYC
Breast, newborn, swollen after injury
    ARN, HEP
  painful CALC, CON
    during pregnancy BRY, CON
    stitching SANG
Breastborn, pain over CACT
Breath, offensive MERC
  shortness while lying ARS
Breathing, labored IP
  shortness of ARS-I, STROP
    on exertion CALC, IOD
Brooding, over imaginary troubles
    NAJA
Bruised feeling ARN, RUTA
Bruises ARN, BEL-P, HAM
Brunettes BRY, NUX-V
Burning pain ARS, PHOS
Burns CAPS
  blistered CANTH, HAM
  infected HEP
  simple URT-U
  ulcerated KALI-BI
  xray X-RAY
Busyness from sexual
    repression LIL-T

Calves, cramps during pregnancy
    COFF, CUP-A, FERR, NUX-V
Carried, babies improve only
    when CHAM

Cautious CALC-C
Chagrin, complaint from
    PH-AC, STAPH
Changing position constantly
    from pain RUTA
  symptoms PUL
Changing weather worsens
    DULC, HYPER, RHOD, TUB
Chest, constricting pain of CACT
  empty sensation STAN
  heaving of RHUS-T
  pain CARB-V
    pricking BRY
    rattling BELL, SUL, TART
    expectoration improves SUL
    with cough HEP
  tighteness of IP
  weakness STAN
    on talking DIG
Chicken pox, after fever has passed
    MERC
  anxiety after COFF
  complication VARIC
  fever ACON
Chicken pox, restlessness of COFF
Childbirth, complaints after SEP
  before ARN
  eased ARIST, CALC-FL
  fear CALEN
Chilliness ALUM, ARG-N, ARS,
    ARS-I, AUR, CALC,
    CARB-AN, GELS, HEP, LED,
    MAG-C, MERC, NUX-V, PSOR,
    SEP, SIL
  after cold wind SEP
  extreme ARS-A, PSOR, VERAT
  shivering from CINCH, MERC
  with cold perspiration TAB
Cholera VERAT
Circulation poor CARB-AN
Closed room worsens PULS
Clothing, averse to CROT-CAS, LACH
Coccyx, pain from falls on HYPER
Coffee worsens NUX-V

Cold drinks, worsen ARS, STAPH
    when overheated ARS
    improves FERR-P
Cold places worsens DULC
Cold, sensitive to HEP
Cold, preventative CALC-C,
    BACIL, NAT-M
    weather worsens DULC
    worsens HYPER, RHUS-T, SEP, SIL
Colds, EUCAL
    after chill ACON, CAMPH
    chilled feet SIL
    exposure to cold CON
    frequent SEP, TUB
    from open air TUB
Colic from green food ARS, COLCH
    in infants MERC, NUX-V
        from anger CHAM
            exposure to cold CHAM
            fatty foods IP, PULS
            worms CINA
        with gas PULS
        with vomiting PULS
Collapse VERAT
Complaining HEP
Concussion, from injury HYPER
Confused, CALC, GELS
Constipation ALUM,
    GRAPH, IGN, IOD,
    NAT-M, NUX-V, SEP, SUL
    alternating with diarrhea NUX-V
    desire for stool absent BRY,OP
    from painful stool SUL
        traveling COC-I
        weariness COC-I
    with unsuccessful desire for stool
Contradiction, cannot endure
    CON, LYC
    worsens LYC
Convulsions, before measles eruption
    CALC
Coordination, muscular, lack of
    GELS

Cough CINCH
    after exposure to colds DULC
        damp DULC
    as if tearing the larynx ALL-C
    barking BELL
    choking HEP
    chronic PHOS
    convulsive CARB-V, DROS
    cold air worsens PHOS
    drinks worsen SPONG
    croupy HEP KALI-BI
    day and night CHAM
    daytime EUPHR, HEP
    drafts worsen SPONG
    drinking worsens PHOS
    dry ACON, BELL, BRY,
        CHAM, HEP, IP,
        MERC, NUX-V, SUL
    eating worsens PHOS
    evening in bed STAN
        worsens CARB-V
    fatiguing IP, NUX-V
    frequent ACON, BRY
    from cold winds ACON
        drafts ACON
      dry winds ACON
    hacking ARS-I
    hoarse CHAM
    hollow BELL
    in chubby children KALI-BI
    influenzal EUCAL
    laughing worsens PHOS, STAN
    loose PULS
    lying improves BRY
        on left side worsens PHOS
        worsens DROS, SPONG
    moist EUPHR
    motion improves DROS
        worsens BRY
    night worsens BELL, CON,
        EUPHR
    paroxysms IP, NUX-V
    of three STAN

Cough (cont'd.)
  reading worsens PHOS
  short ACON
  singing worsens STAN
  south wind worsens EUPHR
  talking worsens PHOS, STAN
  tobacco smoke worsens EUPHR
  violent MERC
  warm drinks worsen STAN
    room worsens BRY
  west wind worsens HEP
  whooping IP
    bad effects of PERT
  wind worsens SPONG
  with asthma SPONG
    gagging BRY, EUPHR
Critical of others LYC
Crying, see *Weeping*
Cursing LIL-T
Cuts BELL

Dampness worsens, DULC, GELS,
    HYPER
Daytime worsens MED
Death, desires own NAJA
Delicate women XANT
Delirious OP
Delusion of being fatally ill PSOR
Depression ARS, BAPT, CALC,
    GELS, LIL-T, SEP, VALER
  after fright HYPER
    operations HYPER
  before menses PHOS, SEP
  emotional, after injuries
        or operations HYPER
Despair ARS, CALC, IGN, LIL-T,
    PSOR
Desires fresh air PULS, SUL
  things immediately BRY
Desires to be left alone GELS
  unobtainable things BRY
Despondent TAB

Diaper rash, in chilly babies CALC,
    HEP
  hot babies SUL
  restless, feverish babies ACON, CHAM
Diarrhea, ALOE, CHAM, COLOC
    PHOS, TAB
  after cold drinks or food
        in hot weather ARS
    drinking ARS, CINCH
    eating ARS, CINCH
Diarrhea, alternates with constipation
    BRY, LACH, NUX-V
  bathing, during PODO
  before menses VERAT
  black LACH
  blood-streaked IP
  bloody COLOC
  chronic PODO, SUL
  cold weather causes IP, MERC,
    NUX-V
  early morning PODO
  eating, after PODO
  foul-smelling like decayed flesh
    PSOR
  from sugar ARG-N
  in children ARG-N
    teething children PODO
  like chopped spinach ARG-N
  night worse ARS, CINCH
  pain, burning ARN
    stool relieves COLOC
  painless ARS, PODO, SUL
  profuse with vomiting VERAT
  protracted SUL
  slimy NUX-V
  slimy green CHAM
  smelly CHAM
  sticky LACH
  strange food causes IP
  two a.m., at ARS
  warm weather causes BRY
  white LACH
  with cough TART

Diarrhea (cont'd.)
  with cough (cont'd.)
    teething MERC, SUL
    vomiting IP
Dirty SUL
Discoloration, bluish, of affected
    parts CROT-H
Disinterested in business CON
  everything AMBR-GR, CON,
    PH-AC, VERAT
Dislocations RUTA
Dissatisfied with whatever offered
    BRY, STAP
Dizziness GELS, TAB
  on closing the eyes TAB
Domineering CON
Drafts, cold, worsens PSOR
Dreams, of death CROT-H
  the dead CROT-H
Dryness ALUM
Dying, feeling as if DIG

Ears, coldness VERAT
  glands below and in front inflamed
    ARN, DULC
  inflamed PULS, SUL
  oozing behind TUB
  pain in cold wind SEP
  swollen shut URT-V
  veins swollen DIG
Eczema, bran-like TUB
  creases of extremities SEP
  dry SEP
  itching SEP
    at night TUB
    while undressing TUB
  summer improves SEP
  wet CAL-C
  white TUB
  winter worsens SEP
Emaciated ARS, IOD
Emotional excitement, complaints
    from GEL
Emotionally passive SIL
Envy worsens STAPH

Epididymis inflamed ARIST
Epilepsy, after injury ARN, NAT-S
  as if dead after OP
Erections, absent AGN-C
  after sexual excesses PHOS-AC
  excessive CALC-P
  long lasting PIC-AC
  painful after injury ARN
  poor LYC
Erections poor after spinal injury
    HYPER
  violent PIC-AC
Evening worsens KALI-S, SEP
Excitable HYOS
Exertion worsens ARS-I, LAT-M
Exhausting diseases, effects of
    CARB-V
Exhaustion DIG
  from bleeding CALEN
    pain CALEN
Expression, drunken BAPT
  hang dog PHOS
  stupid BAPT
Extremities alternately hot and cold
    RHUS-T
  cold CARB-V, CHAM, COLOC,
    SEP
  coldness to touch VERAT
  cracking when stretched THUJ
  numbness LYC
    where lain upon RHUS-T
  stiff BRY
  stretching frequently THUJ
  swelling of APIS
  swollen after heart disease BLAT
    infection APOC
Eyeballs, pain from bruises SYMPH
  sore EUP
Eyelids, burning SABAD
  discolored, red SABAD
  upper, swollen KALI-C
  veins, swollen DIG
Eyes, blue circles around ARS,
    PHOS
    under PHOS

Eyes, bruising injuries to   LED
  burning   ALL-C
  discharge, bland   EUPHR
    irritating   ALL-C
  discoloration from injury   LED
  half-closed   OP
  inflammation   ACON, EUPH, SUL
    after injury   ARN
    cold worsens   RHUS-T
    damp worsens   RHUS-T
    in newborn   ACON, ARG-N, SUL
      improved by activity   RHUS-
    of conjunctiva   HAM-V
  redness of   ACON
  running   ALL-C, PULS
Eyes, sensitivity of   ACON
  to light   BELL
  sties,   AUR-M, PUL, STAPH, SUL
  swollen   URT-U
    underneath   APIS
  tearing   ACON, ALL-C
    morning on rising   EUPHR
  watering   BELL, SABAD

Face, acne,   CARB-B, GRAPH, HEP,
  KALI-BI, SEP, SUL, TUB
  cheeks sunken   ARS
  cold CARB-V
  discoloration, dark   BAPT,
    CROT-H
  earthy complexion   NAT-M
  eruption, crusty, at teething
    RHUS-T
    discharging, irritating   MEZ
    eruption, dry, with teething
      CALC
    eyebrows with teething   SUL
    oozing with teething   LYC
    pustules at teething   ACON,
      VIOL
    red patches in new born   ACON,
      ARN, ANT-C, SEP
  hot   SABAD
  pale   ARS, CALC, CARB-V, IP,
    PHOS, PSUR, TUB

Face (cont'd.)
  perspiring   CARB-V
  pinched   CARB-V
  red   ACON, CHAM, GLON, SUL
    and pale alternate   ACON
    dark   BAPT
  sallow   SEP
  shriveled looking   ARG-N
  sickly   PSOR
Face, swollen   CHAM
  wizened   PHOS
Faintness   DIG, SPONG
  after stool   ALOE
  before lunch   SUL
    menses   NAT-M
  on least exertion   VERAT
Falls   ARN
Fanned, desires to be   CARB-V
Fanning improves   CARB-V
Fatigue   CARB-V, NUX-M
Fatness   CALC-C
Fatty foods worsen   CARB-V, PULS
Fear   CACT, CALC, LIL-T
  after midnight   ARS
Fear before exams   SIL
  being alone   LYC
    observed by others   CALC
  business failure   PSOR
  complaints from   HYPER
  dark   CALC-C
  death   ACON, ARS, CACT, PSOR
  disaster   CALC
  disease   CALC
    is incurable   ARS, PSOR
  dying by inability to breathe
    LAT-M
  everything   PSOR
  future   PSOR
  going out in public   ARG-N
  insanity   CALC
  religious salvation   PSOR
  seasickness   ACON
  thunder   PHOS, RHOD
Feet, chilliness   SIL
Fever   ACON
  alternation with chills   MERC

Fickle PULS
Fidgety PHOS
Fierceness, from sunstroke BELL
Fingernails, discolored blue
   CROT-H
Fingers cracked in winter SEP
   fall asleep DIG
   heaviness STROPH
   joints swollen CAL-F
Flanks bloated NUX-V
Flatus LYC
   burning ALOE
   improved CINCH
   loud CARB-V, LYC, NUX-V
   offensive ALOE
   painful NUX-V
   smelly CARB-V, LYC
      like rotten eggs, SUL
Fog worsens HYPER
Food, fatty, worsens PULS
   tastes sour LYC
Foot, ball of, pain shooting
      RHUS-V
         painful, soreness MED
   bones of, pain, shooting RHUS-V
   heel, pains RHUS-V
   pain, cramping, nighttime CALC
Forearms, heaviness of STROPH
Forehead, cold perspiration of
   VERAT
Fresh air, improves PULS
Fretful NUX-V
   infants CHAM
   menses, during CHAM

Gagging with asthma IP
      cough BRY, EUPHR
Gasping in pain LAT-M
Gassy ARG-N, CARB-V, CINCH,
      COLCH, LYC, NUX-V
   after eating ARG-N, LYC, NUX-V
   from rectum CINCH
Gastric complaints from cold drinks
      on hot days KALI-BI

Gay and sad alternately PLAT
Genitalia sensitive to touch PLAT
Genital itching before menses
   GRAPH
Gentle PULS
Gloomy PHOS
Gonorrhea ARIST
Grief AUR, IGN, PH-AC, STAPH
   from unhappy love affairs PH-AC
Groin pain BORAX
   during menses BORAX
Gums sore MERC

Hair dull SEP
   falling ARS, MERC, NAT-M,
      SEP
   rough ANT-C
   stringy SEP
Hands, numbness LYC
Happiness alternates with sadness
   ARIST
Haughty PLAT
Hay Fever PSOR
   fall worsens ALL-C
   from cold DULC
      heat NAT-M
      sun NAT-M
      wading in cold water DULC
      weather changing hot to cold
         DULC
      wet weather DULC
   previous history of asthma
         or eczema PSOR
   returns yearly at same time
      PSOR
   spring worsens ALL-C
Headache BELL, CINCH, CYCL,
      TAB
   air, open, improves ALL-C
   band-like, around the head GELS
   dull, evening worsens ALL-C
      open air improves ALL-C
      warm room worsens ALL-C
   during menses GEL

Headache (cont'd.)
  early morning TAB
  from hunger LYC
    spinal injury HYPER
    sunrise to sunset GLON
  heat worsens GLON
  jarring worsens GLON
  pulsating GLON
  stepping worsens GLON
  throbbing GLON
Head, bones, brittleness in children
    CALC-P
  thinness in children CALC-P
  fontanelles, closing delayed
    CALC-P
    reopen after closing CALC-P
    swollen CALC, SIL, SUL
  forehead, cold perspiration
    VERAT-A
  hot, BELL, SUL
  perspiration of CALC
    at night CALC
      soaking the pillow CALC
  pressing outwards, sensation of
    ACON
  pulsation of BELL
  swollen feeling GLON
  top of, warmth of ACON
Hearing, weak CARB-AN
Heart action, excited NAJA,
    STROPH
  weak ARS-I
  disease, organic ARS-I
  enlarged NAJA
  failure STROP
  heaving NAJA
  pain SPONG
    cold weather worsens SPIG
    compressing SPIG
    constricting SPONG
    cramping NAJA
    extending to left neck NAJA

Heart action (cont'd.)
    shoulder NAJA
    extending to left LAT-M
      arm LAT-M
      shoulders LAT-M
    lying on left side worsens NAJA
    motion worsens SPIG
    open air improves NAJA
    severe LAT-M, SPIG
    sticking NAJA, SPIG
    twisting TAB
    wet weather worsens SPIG
Heart palpitations IOD, SPONG,
    TAB
  audible SPIG
  violent SPIG
  squeezed rapidly as if IOD
  turning over in chest, sensation of
    CROT-T
  valves weak DIG
  weakness CROT-H
    from previous disease NAJA
    feeling of NAJA
Heartburn of pregnancy CAPS,
    PULS
Heat flashes SEP, SUL
  in evening SUL
  menopausal SEP
Heat worsens APIS, IOD, KALI-BI,
    KALI-S, LACH, MED,
    NAT-M, SUL
Heated, feels SUL
Hemorrhoids AESC, ALOE,
    NIT-AC, NUX-V, SUL
  bathing worsens SUL
  bleeding ALOE
    on touch NIT-AC
  blue grapes, like AESE, ALOE
  burning AESC, SUL
  cold air improves SUL
    bathing improves NUX-V
  constipation, from NUX-V
  hot ALOE

Hemorrhoids (cont'd.)
  itching ALOE, NUX-V, SUL
    scratching worsens SUL
  painful, after stool NIT-AC
    cold water improves ALOE
    like needles NIT-AC
  protrude during urination MUR-AC
  recurrent SUL
  sore ALOE
  standing worsens SUL
  tender ALOE
    on least touch MUR-AC
Hepatitis CHEL
Hips, pain, aching, severe AESC
Hives PULS
Homesickness PH-AC
Homosexuality, female NAT-M, SEP
  male PHOS
Hopeless ARS, AUR, CALC, IGN,
    LIL-T, PSOR
  after midnight ARS
Hostility, suppressed, worsens STAPH
Hot, feels SUL
Hurry, pointless LIL-T
Hypnotism, complaints from HYPER
Hypochondrical HEP

Immobilized ACON, OP
  by fear CALC
Impatient BRY
Impressionable, menses, during CHAM
Indifferent to everything AGN-C,
    ARS, CALC, NUX-M, PH-AC,
    PHOS
  loved ones SEP
Indigestion SIL
  of pregnancy CALC-F
Indignation STAPH
Indolence SEP
Indoors worsens EUPHR
Infections heal slowly SIL
Inflammation after injuries CALEN
Influenza CINCH, EUCAL, EUP
  in horses, MERC, SUL

Influenza (cont'd.)
  prevention ARS, CAD-M
Inhaling, grunting BRY
Injuries ARN
  crushing HYPER
  feel cold to the touch LED
  from falls HAM-V
    sharp instruments STAPH
  infected HEP
Intellectuals LYC, NUX-V
Intense people BRY, NUX-V
Intercourse painful PLAT, SEP,
    STAPH
Intestinal colic from bad food ARS
    constipation ARS, NUX-V
    drinking cold water ARS
Introversion SIL
Irritable ARS, BRY, CACT, CHAM,
    HEP, LYC, NAT-M, NUX-V,
    SEP, SUL, VALER
  before menses KREOS, MAG-M,
  SEP

Jarring, sensitive to HYPER, LED
Jealousy, complaints from APIS, HYOS
Joints cracking MED, NAT-M, SEP
  fluid lost by penetrating wounds
    CALEN
  hot BRY
  pains CINCH, FER-P
    climbing stairs worsens CALC
    cold weather worsens RHUS-T
    drafts worsens RHUS-T
    eating worsens CALC
    pains, gouty BRY
    heat improves RHUS-T, SEP
     worsens KALI-S, LYC
    massage improves RHUS-T
    menopausal SEP
    motion, continued, improves
     RHUS-T
     improves LYC, RHUS-T
     on first, RHUS-T

Joints (cont'd.)
  pains (cont'd.)
    motion (cont'd.)
      worsens BRY, CALC,
        FERR-P
      nighttime RHUS-T
      rest worsens LYC
      shifting from place to place
        KALI-S, MED
      sided, left SEP
        right LYC
      stinging BRY
        on standing NAT-M
        walking NAT-M
      tearing on standing NAT-M
        walking NAT-M
      water worsens CALC
      wet weather worsens RHUS-T
    redness BRY
    sprained by slight exertion
      CARB-AN
    stiff BRY, SEP
      morning, on rising RHUS-T
      walking MED
    swollen, BRY, KALI-S
    tender, BRY
    weakness CARB-AN
      profound SEP

Kidney disease ACON
    from exposure to dampness
      DULC
      injury ARN

Lameness ARN
Laughing easily PULS
Legs, aching CINCH
  calves, cramps at night CALC
  drawn against abdomen CHAM
  eruptions, oozing SUL, THUJ
    itching SUL, THUJ
    scurfy, SUL, THUJ
  heels, eruptions, red, flat ARS,
    SEC, THUJ

Legs (cont'd.)
  heels (cont'd.)
    ulcers MERC
  swollen, watery, cold to touch
    CINCH
    hot ACON, RHUS-T
    painful ACON
    stiff RHUS-T
  weakness before menses COLC
Life a burden AUR
Limbs, aching BAPT
  motion worsens BRY
  cold, wet CALC
  jerking, sudden BELL
  moving constantly CHAM, OP
Lips, cracked BRY
  dry BRY
  picking at ARUM-T
  swollen shut URT-V
  upper, inflamed ARUM-T
  veins swollen DIG
Listless LIL-T, PHOS-AC
Loins, dragging KALI-C
  weakness KALI-C
Lying left side worsens NAJA
  painful side improves BRY
  right side worsens CROT-H

Mange, HEP, NAT-M, PSOR,
  SEP, SUL
Masturbation, excessive, BUFO,
  ORIG, PH-AC, PHOS
Measles, PULS
  complications of MORB
  fever, ACON, SUL
  rash ANT-T
    burning afterward ARS, SUL
    itching ARS, SUL
  suppressed by cold, followed by
    respiratory conditions BRY
    chest affected PHOS
    diarrhea follows PULS
    vomiting follows ARS, CHAM,
      IP

Measles (cont'd.)
  skin tender after RHUS-T
Melancholy before menses CAUS,
    LYC
Memory, poor AUR, BAR-C,
    CARB-V, CON, NUX-M
  for familiar things NUX-M
Menopause GRAPH, LACH, SEP
Menses
  absent ARIST, SUL
    due to chill ACON
  before, worsened ARIST, SEP
  between, worsened BELL
  black, MAG-C, PULS
    clots CINCH
    shreds CROC
  bright red FICUS, IP, SABIN
  clotted, PULS, SEP, THALAS
    dark PLAT
  colicky BORAX
  cramping pain VIBUR
  dark HAM, SEC
  delayed ARIST, MAG-C, SUL
    in young girls CYCL, PULS
  difficult from injuries to
      coccyx HYPER
  early ALOE, BORAX, CALC,
    PLAT, XANT
  excessive, ARS, USTIL
    after anger CHAM
    irritation CHAM
  fluid SEC
  frequent SEP
  hemorrhage, like a THALS
  increased FER
  infrequent SEP
  intermittent in young girls PULS
  irregular SENEC, SEP
  long, SEP
  night worsens MAG-C
  offensive BELL
  painful CHAM, SENEC, XANT
    hot application relieve MAG-P

Menses (cont'd.)
  painful (cont'd.)
    in attacks MAG-P
      in young girls GELS
    make her cry out CACT
  paroxysmal SABIN
  profuse BORAX, CALC-C,
    FICUS, PLAT, SEP, XANT
  prolonged ARIST, SEP
  scanty, CON, NAT-M, PULS,
    SENEC, SEP, SUL
  short ARIST, SEP
  standing improves SABIN
  suppressed from being chilled ACON
    wet feet PULS
  tarry MAG-C
  thin SEP
  unendurable pain with ACON
  walking improves SABIN
  worse before SEP
Midnight, after, worsens ARS
Mild PULS
Milk worsens TUB
Mind, dullness of ACON
  tiredness of, from overwork ARG-N
Miscarriage SEP
  first three months SEP
  threatened PULS, SEP
Moods alternate LIL-T
  swing wildly NUX-M
Moon, new, worsens ALUM
  full ALUM
Morning sickness NUX-V, SEP
    after fats PULS
    fresh air improves PULS
    in gassy persons CALC-F
  worse in LACH, NUX-V, STAPH
Mortification, complaints from
    STAPH
Motion, continued, improves
    RHUS-T
  sensitive to HYPER LED
  slow VERAT

Motion (cont'd.)
  worsens BRY, FER-P, MED,
    NUX-V
Mouth, dry, ACON, BRY, PULS
  salivation IP
  ulcers, MERC
Mucous, stringy KALI-BI
  tough KALI-BI
  viscid KALI-BI
Mumps BELL, MERC
  complications PAROT
Muscles, not obey will GELS
  ruptured CALEN
  strained on lifting smallest weight
    CARB-AN

Nails, malformed, twisted SIL
Nausea, BOR, IP, PULS, STROP, TAB
  after drinking APOC
    eating NUX-V
    meals NUX-V
  air cold, improves TAB
    fresh TAB
  at smell of food CINCH, SEP
  before menses VERAT
  constant IP
  eating worsens NUX-V
  morning NUX-V
  motion of cars SEP
    worsens TAB
  of pregnancy, continuous PETR,
    TAB
      from motion SEP
      morning SEP
      with retching SYMP
  on descending BOR
    motion APOM, BOR
    sight of boat in motion COC-C
  riding in vehicle COC-C
  vomiting relieves NUX-V
Neck glands swollen MERC
Nerve injuries HYPER LED

Nerve tumors CALEND
Nervousness IGN, ACT-R, VERAT
Night improves MED
  2 a.m. worsens ARS, BELL, CALC
Nipples, burning SANG
  sore SANG
Nose, as if worms crawling inside
  NAT-M
  discharge ALL-C, SABAD
    acrid ALL-C, ARUM-T
    bland ALL-C
    burning ALL-C
    colored PULS
    foul EUCAL
    irritating ALL-C, EUCAL,
      EUPHR
    morning on rising EUPHR
    plugs KALI-BI
    profuse ALL-C, ARUM-T
      MERC
    thick PULS
    watery ALL-C, MERC
  discoloration, greenish-yellow over
    bridge SEP
  inflamed ARUM-T, RHUS-T
  pain on touch RHUS-T
  picking ARUM-T, CINA
  red RHUS-T
  running ACON, EUP
  soreness MERC
Nose, swollen shut URT-V
Not finish projects SIL
Numbness IGN

Obese PULS
Obscene speech LIL-T
Odor, sour MAG-C
Old looking AGN-C, ARG-N
Open air improves ARS-I, PULS
  worsens CYCL
Operations, before ARN
  effects of ARN, STAPH

Opposition, cannot endure   LYC
Ovaries, painful   HAM
   during menses   BELL
   following injuries to coccyx
   HYPER
Oversensitive to pain   IGN

Pain, aching   GELS
  bearing-down before menses
    MAG-C, SEP
  burning like fire   ARS
  cold improves   LED
  cuffing   STAPH
  shifting   PULS
  smarting   STAPH
  stinging   STAPH
Painful parts, cold worsens   BRY
   lying on improves   BRY
   perspiration improves   BRY
   touch worsens   BRY
Palpitations, frequent   AUR
Parts rested on feel sore BAPT,
   RUTA
Peevish,   CHAM, LYC
Pelvic organs, as if falling out   SEP
   heat of ascending   SEP
Pelvis, pain, bearing down,   ALOE,
   FICUS, NIT-AC
   cramping   CHAM, VIBUR
People, aversion to   CHAM
Periodocity   CINCH
  7-14 days worsen   CINCH
  14 days worsen   ALUM
  worse at same time each day   CEDR
Perspiration SPONG
  cold,   CACT, CARB-V, TAB
   with chilliness   TAB
  excessive   MERC
  night   MERC
  odor, foul   CINCH
  profuse   CACT, CALC, CINCH,
    MERC

Perspiration (cont'd.)
  profuse (cont'd.)
    after slight exertion   CALC
    and hot   OP
    night   MERC
Piles, see *Hemorrhoids*
Plunges, downward,   XERAT
Poison ivy protection   RHUS-T
Poisonous bites   LED
Pollution, air   SULFS-AC
Pressure   LACH
Pride worsens   PLAT, STAPH
Prostration, extreme   DIG
  profound,   ARS, TAB, VERAT
Prostate, inflamed   ARIST
Public appearances, worse before   LYC
Pulse, frequent,   ARS, LAT-M,
   STROP
  irregular   ARS, BELL, SPIG
   intensity   NAJA
   rate   STROP
  rapid   ACON, VERAT
  slow   DIG
  weak,   CACT, CAMPH, LAT-M,
   STROP

Quarrelsome   CON, NUX-V
Quitters   SIL

Rage, suppressed, worsens   STAPH
Rectum, dry   AESC
Respiration, difficult   BELL
  fast,   ACON, BELL, BRY
  gasping   SPONG
  hot   ACON
  labored   BRY, OP
  stertorous   OP
  wheezing during cough   CUPR-A
Restless,   ACON, ARG-N, ARS,
   BELL, CHAM, COLOC, IP,
   LIL-T, RHUS-T,   SUL

Restless (cont'd.)
 after midnight ARS
 emotional ACON
 extreme ARS
 menses, before KREOS
  during ACT-R
 physical ACON, RHUS-T, SUL
Rheumatism, acute DULC
Right side worse LYC

Sadness AGN-C, CALC, PSOR,
  SEP, STAN
 alternates with happiness ARIST
 during menses ACT-R
Salivation, profuse CINCH, MERC
Sallowness SEP
Scalp, oozing of TUB
Scarlet fever, BELL, MERC, NUX-V,
  OP, PULS, SUL
Scrawny (thin) NAT-M
Seashore improves MED
 worsens NAT-M
Seasickness COLC
 during menses COLC
Secretions increased STROP
Self-contempt AGN-C
Sensitive PHOS, STAPH
 emotionally STAPH
 extreme HEP
 sensitive to:
  alcohol NUX-V
  coffee NUX-V
  criticism NUX-V
  emotional hurt STAPH
  everything NUX-V, PHOS
  lights NUX-V, NUX-M, PHOS
  mental exertion NUX-V
  music NUX-V
  noise, NUX-M, NUX-V, PHOS
  odors, NUX-M, NUX-V, PHOS
  people NUX-V
  slight HEP

Sensitive (cont'd.)
 sensitive to (cont'd.)
  spices NUX-V
  tobacco smoke NUX-V
  touch, NUX-M, NUX-V,
   PHOS, SPIG
Sexual desire ARIST
 excessive CALC-P, PHOS,
  PIC-AC
  in women ORIG, PLAT
 lost SEP
 suppressed, complaints from CON
Shivering MERC
Shock, complaints from HYPER
Shoulder, discoloration, right BRY
 pain, MED, RHUS-T
  left side MED
  right, extending to upper arm BRY
Shoulders, stiff, as if sprained
  RHUS-T
 swelling, right BRY
Shy, SIL
Sided, left, worsens LACH, LIL-T
  SEP
 right worsens LYC
Sighing, involuntary IGN
Sinus trouble KALI-BI
Sitting uncomfortable as things feel
  hard ARN
Skin, black and blue bruises LED
 blisters, watery SEP
  whitish SEP
 blue CARB-V, DIG
 burning in spots PULS
Skin, chafing in infants ARN,
  CHAM, LYC, MERC, SUL,
 cold and clammy CALC
  to touch VERAT-A
 conditions ARIST
 discoloration, pale CALC
  red spots PULS
  sallow SEP

Skin (cont'd.)
  dry   ACON, BELL, PULS,
        SABAD
  eruption   CARB-V, PULS, SUL
    cool bathing improves   PULS
    from eating fats   PULS
      pork   PULS
    itching   URT-V
  flabby   ARS
  folds ooze   TUB
  hard patches   ARS, RHUS-T, THUJ
  hot   ACON, PULS, URT-U
  icy cold to touch   CAMPH, VERAT
  infected easily   SIL
  inflammation   RHUS-T
  leaden color in bald spots   MERC
  loose   ARS
  numbness   URT-U
  odor, fishy   SEP
    rotten eggs   SUL
  oily   SEP
  pale   DIG
  patches, raised   RHUS-T
  pimples   THUJ
  prickling   PULS
    heat   ACON, BRY, CHAM, SUL
  pustules inflamed   ACON
  ring worm   RHUS-T, SEP, SUL
  rough scales   ANT-C
  scabs   RHUS-T
 · scurfy patches   ARS
  sensitive to least touch   LACH
  tender when touched   SEP
  tingling   URT-U
  troubles   TUB
  ulcers with hard, red edges   ARN
  yellow in newborn   CINCH, MERC
Sleep, after, worsened   LACH
  interrupted by cold, extremities
        CARB-V
Sleepiness early in evening
        NUX-V, SUL
  overpowering   NUX-M
Sleepless   ARS, BELL, VALER
  all night, sleepy in daytime   STAPH

Sneezing   ACON, BELL, PULS
  follows cough   BELL
  paroxysms   SABAD
  peaches, handling worsens   ALL-C
  rising worsens   ALL-C
Society, avoids   CON
Soreness   ARN
Sour disposition   MAG-C
Speech difficult from weariness   COC-I
  slowly answers   PHOS
  weak during menses   CARB-AN
  words misplaced   CALC
  wrong words in   NUX-M
Spine, injuries to   HYPER
Spit   CHAM
  bloody   NAT-M
  expelled   easily DULC
  green   SUL
  greenish-yellow   STAN
  lumpy   SUL
  profuse   STAN
  salty   STAN
  sweet   STAN
Sprains   ARN, BEL-P, LED,
        RHUS-T, RUTA
  cold worsens   CALC, RHUS-T,
        RUTA
  damp worsens   CALC, RHUS-T,
        RUTA
  exercise improves   RHUS-T, RUTA
    worsens   CALC
  pain of, extends to bones   RUTA
  rest worsens   RHUS-T, RUTA
  warmth improves   CALC,
        RHUS-T, RUTA
Staggering   VERAT
  on motion of the head   GELS
Standing worsens   SUL
Sterility   ARIS, SEP
Stiffness   EUCAL
  from long riding   ARN
Stings, bee   APIS, URT-U
  ants   FORM-R
  infected   CANTH
  insects   LED

Stings (cont'd.)
  spiders TARENT
  wasps ARN, VESP
Stomach, burning STROPH
  faint feeling in TAB
  heavy feeling NUX-V
  sinking in DIG, TAB
  upsets ARIST
    from alcohol, coffee or tobacco
      NUX-V
      cold drinks BRY
      spicy foods NUX-V
  vomiting with cough IP, NUX-V
Stool, dark BRY, OP
  dry, BRY, OP, SUL
    as if burnt BRY
  foul-smelling ARN, COLOC,
    PODO, SUL
  frequent ARN
  green PODO
  hard OP
    as if burnt SUL
  knotty SUL
  large BRY, SUL
  odor of rotten eggs CHAM
  painful SUL
  profuse PODO
  putrid IP
  slimy ARN
  sour odor MERC
  spottering COLOC
  urging to ALOE
  watery MERC, PODO
  worms CINA
Storm before, worsens, RHOD
Striking at others LIL-T
Stroke from heat GLON
Stubborn SÍL
Stuffy room worsens APIS, PULS,
  SUL
Stupid feeling ACON
Stupor BAPT, PHOS
Suffocating sensation SPONG
Suicidal AUR, PSOR
Sun worsens GLON, MED,

Sun worsens (cont'd.)
  NAT-M, SUL
Sweat cold TAB
Swelling, after Bright's disease DIG
  after scarlet fever DIG
  red FER-P, RHUS-T
  shiny RHUS-T
  smooth RHUS-T
  warmth worsens APIS

Taste, bitter, NUX-V
  foul PULS
  sour NAT-M, NUX-V
    with heartburn CALC
Tears, irritating ALL-C
Teething ACON, CHAM, COFF
  complicated CALC, CHAM
  delayed CALC-P
Tendons, ruptured CALEN
Testicles, inflamed in mumps PULS
Tests, worse before LYC
Thighs, pain in NIT-AC
Thin ALUM, ARG-N, IOD-M,
  NAT-M, NUX-V
Thinking, poor NUX-V
  slow CARB-V, PHOS-AC, PULS
Thirsty ACON, APOC, ARS, BELL,
  BRY, COLOC, PULS
Thirst for cold water in small sips ARS
  excessive ANT-C
  extreme BRY
  for cold drinks ACON, SUL
    ice cold water VERAT
  large, infrequent amounts BRY
  unquenchable BRY
Thirstless PUL
Thoughts vanish while reading,
  talking, or writing NUX-V
Throat, ball, sensation of IGN
  burning STROPH
  dark red BAPT
  dry SABAD
  putrid BAPT
  rattling, during inspiration BELL

Throat (cont'd.)
  splinter sensation on swallowing
    ARG-N
  windpipe painful   PHOS
Thunderstorms worsen   MED,
    PHOS
Timid   LIL-T, PULS
Tiredness   ARN, AUR, BEL-P,
    CALC, CINCH, EUCAL, GELS,
    PH-AC, PHOS, PIC-AC, SEP, SIL,
    THALAS
  from slight exertion   SIL
  so speech impossible   GELS
Tobacco smoke worsens   IGN,
    NUX-V
Toe, discolored red   NAT-M
  swollen NAT-M
Tongue
  coated brown   NUX-V
    white   NUX-V
    yellow   KALI-S
  cracked   BRY
  dry   BRY
  moist and white   PULS
  red   ARS
  tip, red   NUX-V
  veins, swollen   DIG
Touch, sensitive to touch of injured parts
    HYPER, STAPH
  worsens   LACH
Trembling   GELS, VERAT
  from weakness   GELS
Twitching of body   STROPH

Ulcers, bleeding   PHOS
Unconscious from coughing   CUP
Uncovers feet at night   SUL
Unsure of self   SIL
Urethra, burning   CANTH
  inflammation   ARIST
Urination, frequent   APIS, RHUS-T
  in pregnancy   BELL, NUX-V, PULS
  involuntary with cough   VERAT
  irritation   APIS

Urination (cont'd.)
  leaking after coughing   CAUST
  night in bed   SEP, SIL
  pain on   CANTH, HYOS
  painful   CAN-S
    urging   CANTH, HYOS
  profuse   MERC
  retarded   CAN-S
  retention   CANTH, HYOS
  spurting   CAN-S
  urgency, constant   CANTH
  urging, painful after urination
    CANTH
Urine bloody   CANTH
  dark   URT-U
  fiery red   ACON
  muddy deposit   ACON
  profuse   URT-U
  retention, painful,   APIS,
    CANTH, HYOS
  scalding   APIS
  scanty   PUL
  smell offensive   VIOL
    like horse's urine   NIT-AC
  suppressed   DIG
  uric acid crystals   URT-U
Uterus, pain dragging   Mag-C

Vagina bleeding at menopause
    NIT-AC
    menses, after   USTIL
      before   USTIL
    miscarriage, after   NIT-AC
  constriction   PLUMB
  discharge   ARIST
    bright red   IP
    brown   ARIST
    burning   ARS
    corrosive   ARS
    itching   ARIST
    offensive   BELL
  pain from pressure of clothing
    STAPH
    on intercourse   SEP

Vagina (cont'd.)
  slimy ARIST
  thin ARS
Varicose vein ARIST
Vertigo, see *Dizzy*
Vertigo CYCL
  lying down worsens CON
  menses, during COCC
  turning in bed CON
Visual disturbances CYCL
Voice hoarseness ARUM-T, BELL,
    PHOS, PULS
  singing worsens ARUM-T
  talking worsens ARUM-T
  uncertain ARUM-T
  with cough MERC
Vomiting, BELL, IP, CINCH,
    STROPH, TAB
  after cough CUP, DROS, PULS
  after meals FERR
  air, fresh, improves TAB
  blood ARN
  during cough NUX-V
  food when hits stomach NUX-V
  motion worsens TAB
  mucous, shiny, white IP
  night TART
  on riding in a vehicle COCC
  with asthma IP
    diarrhea IP, VERAT
    profuse diarrhea, VERAT

Waking 3-4 a.m. NUX-V
Walking, aversion to LIL-T
  with difficulty GELS
Warmth, feeling of NAT-M
  improves STAPH
  in women IOD
  worsens EUPHR, IOD,LED,
    PULS, SUL

Weak ARS, GELS, IOD, PHOS,
    TAB
  after anemia CARB-V, SEP
    hepatitis CHEL, SUL
    menses VERAT
  before menses MAG-C
    during CARB-AN, VERAT
  from grief PHOS-AC
    worry HYPER
  general CARB-AN
Weakness in children BAR-C, LYC,
    SIL
  muscles CARB-AN, SIL
  old age BAR-C, LYC, NUX-M,
    PHOS-AC
  physical LYC
  profound IOD
  whole body VERAT
  with cough TART
  tubercular family history TUB
Weary of life PHOS
Weakness, extreme COC-I
Weather, cold, worsens ARS-I
  dry, worsens ARS-I
  windy, worsens ARS-I
Weeping BELL, LIL-T, PHOS-AC,
    PULS, SEP, STAN
  after coughing ARN, HEP
  causeless NAT-M
  constant AMBER-GR
    holding improves CHAM
  menses, before SEP
Weight, loss (thin) IOD
Wet packs improve CALC-F
  weather worsens CALC-F, DULC
Wind, cold worsens SEP
Wind worsens PULS, RHOD, SEP
Withdrawn from life PHOS,
    PHOS-AC
Woman, diseases of PULS

USEFUL ADDRESSES

Homoeopathic Hospitals
The following provide facilities within the National Health Service:

The Royal London Homoeopathic Hospital, Great Ormond Street, London WC1N 3HR.
(Tel. 01-837 3091)
The Bristol Homoeopathic Hospital, Cotham Road, Cotham, Bristol BS6 6JU.
(Tel. 0272 33068)
The Glasgow Homoeopathic Hospital, 1000 Great Western Road, Glasgow W2.
(Tel. 041-339 0382)
    Outpatients Department, 5 Lynedoch Crescent, Glasgow C3.
    (Tel. 041-332 4490)
Tunbridge Wells Homoeopathic Hospital, Church Road, Tunbridge Wells, Kent.
(Tel. 0892 25065)

Homoeopathic Chemists

A. Nelson and Co., 73 Duke Street, London W1M 6BY.
(Tel. 01-629 3118)
E. Gould and Sons, 14 Crowndale Road, London NW1.
(Tel. 01-388 4752)
Kilburn Chemists Ltd., 216 Belsize Road, London NW6.
(Tel. 01-328 1030)
Stewarts Pharmacy, 59 Sheen Lane, London SW14.
(Tel. 01-876 1861)
Ainsworth's Homoeopathic Pharmacy, 38 New Cavendish Street, London W1M 7LH.
(Tel. 01-935 5330)
Platt's Chemists, 227 Seaview Road, Wallasey, Merseyside.
(Tel. 051-639 1914)
Weleda (UK) Ltd., Heanor Road, Ilkeston, Derbyshire DE7 8DR.
(Tel. 0602 303151)
Freemans, 7 Eaglesham Road, Clarkston, Glasgow G76 5EV.